Welcome to the **Gastric Bypass Meal Prep Cookbook: 110+ Prep-Ready Recipes for a Healthier You.** This cookbook is designed to be your essential guide for navigating life after gastric bypass surgery, providing you with delicious, nutritious, and convenient meal prep recipes to support your health and wellness journey.

Embracing a New Lifestyle

Gastric bypass surgery is a significant step towards achieving your health and weight loss goals. It comes with unique dietary requirements and a commitment to long-term lifestyle changes. Proper nutrition is crucial in your recovery and ongoing success, and meal prepping can be a game-changer in managing your dietary needs effectively.

Why Meal Prep?

Meal prepping offers numerous benefits, especially for those adjusting to new eating habits post-surgery:

- **Convenience:** Having meals prepared in advance saves time and reduces stress, making it easier to stick to your dietary plan.

- **Portion Control:** Prepping meals helps you manage portion sizes, ensuring you consume the right amount of food without overeating.

- **Nutritional Balance:** Planning and preparing your meals ahead ensures that each meal is nutritionally balanced, meeting your protein, vitamin, and mineral needs.

- **Cost-Effective:** Meal prepping can save money by reducing food waste and minimizing the need for last-minute, often unhealthy, food choices.

What You'll Discover Inside

- **110+ Prep-Ready Recipes:** From breakfast to dinner, snacks to desserts, this cookbook provides a wide variety of recipes that are easy to prepare and store, perfect for your meal prep routine.

- **Nutrient-Dense Ingredients:** Each recipe is crafted with ingredients that are rich in essential nutrients, focusing on high-protein, low-fat, and easily digestible options to support your post-surgery needs.

- **Step-by-Step Instructions:** Clear and concise instructions guide you through the meal prep process, making it accessible for everyone, whether you're new to cooking or an experienced chef.

- ***Practical Tips:*** Learn tips and tricks for efficient meal prepping, including storage solutions, reheating techniques, and ways to keep your meals fresh and delicious throughout the week.

Thank you for choosing this cookbook as your companion on your path to a healthier you. Here's to your success, well-being, and the delicious meals ahead. Happy prepping and bon appétit!

1. Clear Broth (chicken, beef, vegetable)

Ingredients:

- 4 lbs chicken bones, beef bones, or vegetable scraps (onion, carrot, celery)
- 1 onion, roughly chopped
- 2 carrots, roughly chopped
- 2 stalks celery, roughly chopped
- 1 bay leaf
- 1 tsp whole peppercorns
- 1 tsp salt (or to taste)

Instructions:

1. Place the bones/vegetable scraps, onion, carrots, celery, bay leaf, and peppercorns in a large stock pot. Cover with cold water by 2 inches.

2. Bring the pot to a boil over high heat. Once boiling, reduce heat to low and let simmer gently for:
- Chicken: 3•4 hours
- Beef: 6•8 hours
- Vegetable: 1•2 hours

3. Skim any foam or fat that rises to the surface during simmering. Strain the broth through a fine mesh sieve, discarding the solids.

4. Season the broth with salt to taste. Use the broth immediately or let cool completely, then refrigerate for up to 1 week or freeze for up to 3 months.

The long simmering time helps extract maximum flavor and nutrients from the bones/vegetables. This clear broth can be used as a base for soups, stews, or enjoyed on its own.

2. Sugar•free Gelatin

Ingredients:

• 1 (0.25 oz) packet unflavored gelatin powder
• 1 cup unsweetened fruit juice or broth (such as apple, grape, chicken, or beef)

Instructions:

1. Pour the fruit juice or broth into a small saucepan and sprinkle the gelatin powder over the top. Let it sit for 2•3 minutes to bloom and soften the gelatin.

2. Place the saucepan over medium heat and whisk constantly until the gelatin is fully dissolved, about 2•3 minutes. Do not let it boil.

3. Pour the gelatin mixture into individual ramekins, molds, or a baking dish. Refrigerate for at least 4 hours, or until completely set.

4. Once set, the gelatin can be unmolded and served. Top with additional fruit juice, broth, or sugar•free whipped cream if desired.

Tips:
• Use unsweetened fruit juices or broths to keep it sugar•free.

• You can use different juice flavors to change up the taste.

• For a firmer set, use 1.5 packets of gelatin per 1 cup of liquid.

• Refrigerate any leftovers for up to 1 week.

This sugar•free gelatin can be a great way to get fluids and nutrients after gastric bypass surgery when solid foods may be difficult to tolerate. Adjust portion sizes as needed based on your individual dietary needs.

3. Decaffeinated Herbal Tea

Ingredients:

- 1 cup water
- 1 herbal tea bag (caffeine•free)
- Lemon slice or honey (optional)

Instructions:

1. Bring the water to a boil in a small saucepan or kettle.

2. Place the herbal tea bag in a mug or teapot. Pour the boiling water over the tea bag.

3. Allow the tea to steep for 5•7 minutes, or according to the package instructions.

4. Remove the tea bag. You can add a slice of lemon or a small drizzle of honey if desired, but keep in mind that honey does contain some sugar.

Herbal Tea Options:
Some good caffeine•free herbal tea options include:
- Chamomile
- Peppermint
- Ginger
- Rooibos
- Hibiscus
- Lemon verbena

Tips:
- Avoid caffeinated teas, as caffeine can be irritating after gastric bypass.

- Sip the tea slowly to help stay hydrated.

- You can make a larger batch and refrigerate it for easy access throughout the day.

- Adjust the strength of the tea to your personal taste preference.

This decaffeinated herbal tea can be a soothing and hydrating option as part of your gastric bypass meal prep and recovery plan. Be sure to check with your healthcare team for any specific dietary recommendations.

4. Diluted Apple Juice

Ingredients:

• 1 cup unsweetened apple juice
• 1 cup water

Instructions:

1. In a pitcher or container, combine the unsweetened apple juice and water.

2. Stir or whisk the mixture until well combined.

That's it! The diluted apple juice is now ready to serve.

Tips:

• Use 100% pure, unsweetened apple juice. Avoid any apple juice with added sugars.

• The 1:1 ratio of juice to water helps dilute the natural sugars in the apple juice.

• You can adjust the ratio of juice to water to your preference, starting with a higher juice concentration and gradually increasing the water as tolerated.

• Refrigerate the diluted apple juice and consume within 3•4 days.

Reasons for Diluting Apple Juice:

• After gastric bypass surgery, consuming concentrated fruit juices can cause dumping syndrome, where the sugars rapidly enter the small intestine.

• Diluting the juice helps slow the absorption of the sugars, making it easier to tolerate.

• The added water also helps increase fluid intake, which is important for hydration during recovery.

This diluted apple juice can be a good option to include in your gastric bypass meal prep, providing some natural sweetness and nutrients while being easier on the digestive system. As always, check with your healthcare team for any specific dietary recommendations.

5. Diluted Cranberry Juice

Ingredients:

• 1 cup unsweetened cranberry juice
• 1 cup water

Instructions:

1. In a pitcher or container, combine the unsweetened cranberry juice and water.

2. Stir or whisk the mixture until well combined.

That's it! The diluted cranberry juice is now ready to serve.

Tips:

• Use 100% pure, unsweetened cranberry juice. Avoid any cranberry juice with added sugars.

• The 1:1 ratio of juice to water helps dilute the natural sugars in the cranberry juice.

• You can adjust the ratio of juice to water to your preference, starting with a higher juice concentration and gradually increasing the water as tolerated.

• Refrigerate the diluted cranberry juice and consume within 3•4 days.

Reasons for Diluting Cranberry Juice:

• After gastric bypass surgery, consuming concentrated fruit juices can cause dumping syndrome, where the sugars rapidly enter the small intestine.

• Diluting the juice helps slow the absorption of the sugars, making it easier to tolerate.

• The added water also helps increase fluid intake, which is important for hydration during recovery.

• Cranberry juice can also help support urinary tract health, which can be beneficial after surgery.

This diluted cranberry juice can be a good option to include in your gastric bypass meal prep, providing some natural sweetness and nutrients while being easier on the digestive system. As always, check with your healthcare team for any specific dietary recommendations.

6. Diluted Grape Juice

Ingredients:

• 1 cup unsweetened grape juice
• 1 cup water

Instructions:

1. In a pitcher or container, combine the unsweetened grape juice and water.

2. Stir or whisk the mixture until well combined.

That's it! The diluted grape juice is now ready to serve.

Tips:

• Use 100% pure, unsweetened grape juice. Avoid any grape juice with added sugars.

• The 1:1 ratio of juice to water helps dilute the natural sugars in the grape juice.

• You can adjust the ratio of juice to water to your preference, starting with a higher juice concentration and gradually increasing the water as tolerated.

• Refrigerate the diluted grape juice and consume within 3•4 days.

Reasons for Diluting Grape Juice:

• After gastric bypass surgery, consuming concentrated fruit juices can cause dumping syndrome, where the sugars rapidly enter the small intestine.

• Diluting the juice helps slow the absorption of the sugars, making it easier to tolerate.

• The added water also helps increase fluid intake, which is important for hydration during recovery.

• Grape juice contains antioxidants and other beneficial compounds that may support overall health.

This diluted grape juice can be a good option to include in your gastric bypass meal prep, providing some natural sweetness and nutrients while being easier on the digestive system. As always, check with your healthcare team for any specific dietary recommendations.

7. Electrolyte Drinks (sugar•free)

Ingredients:

- 4 cups water
- 1/2 teaspoon salt
- 1/4 teaspoon potassium chloride (salt substitute)
- 1/4 cup lemon or lime juice (or to taste)
- Stevia or other no•calorie sweetener (optional)

Instructions:

1. In a pitcher or large container, combine the water, salt, and potassium chloride. Stir until the salts are fully dissolved.

2. Add the lemon or lime juice and stir to combine. Taste and adjust the amount of juice to your preference.

3. If desired, add a few drops of stevia or other no•calorie sweetener to balance the tartness of the citrus.

4. Refrigerate the electrolyte drink until ready to serve.

Tips:
- The salt and potassium chloride help replace electrolytes that can be lost through vomiting, diarrhea, or excessive sweating after surgery.

- You can use other citrus juices like orange or grapefruit, but avoid juices with added sugars.

- Start with the minimum amounts of salt and potassium chloride and adjust to your taste preferences.

- Drink the electrolyte drink slowly throughout the day to stay hydrated.

- Store any leftovers in the refrigerator for up to 5 days.

This sugar•free electrolyte drink can be a helpful addition to your gastric bypass meal prep, providing hydration and replenishing important minerals. As always, consult with your healthcare team for any specific dietary recommendations.

8. Ice Chips

Ingredients:

• Water

Instructions:

1. Fill ice cube trays or small silicone molds with water.

2. Place the trays or molds in the freezer and freeze until solid, about 2•4 hours.

3. Once frozen, pop the ice cubes out of the trays or molds.

4. Break or crush the ice cubes into smaller, chip•like pieces.

5. Store the ice chips in an airtight container or resealable plastic bag in the freezer.

Tips:

• You can use plain water or try flavoring the water with a small amount of unsweetened fruit juice, herbal tea, or a splash of lemon or lime juice before freezing.

• Avoid adding any sweeteners, as that can be difficult to tolerate after gastric bypass.

• Suck on the ice chips slowly to help stay hydrated and soothe any mouth or throat discomfort.

• Ice chips can provide a refreshing and hydrating option when solid foods are difficult to tolerate.

• Adjust the size of the ice chips based on your comfort and ability to swallow.

• Store the ice chips in the freezer for up to 2•3 months.

Ice chips can be a great addition to your gastric bypass meal prep, providing a way to stay hydrated and soothe any discomfort during the recovery process. As always, consult with your healthcare team for any specific dietary recommendations.

9. Popsicles (sugar•free)

Ingredients:

• 2 cups unsweetened fruit juice or pureed fruit (such as apple, grape, berry, or citrus)
• 1/4 cup water
• 1 packet unflavored gelatin powder

Instructions:

1. In a small saucepan, sprinkle the gelatin powder over the fruit juice or pureed fruit. Let it sit for 2•3 minutes to bloom.

2. Place the saucepan over medium heat and whisk constantly until the gelatin is fully dissolved, about 2•3 minutes. Do not let it boil.

3. Remove the saucepan from the heat and stir in the 1/4 cup of water until well combined.

4. Carefully pour the mixture into popsicle molds, leaving a small amount of headspace at the top for expansion.

5. Freeze the popsicles for at least 4 hours, or until completely set.

6. To remove the popsicles, run the molds under warm water for a few seconds, then gently pull the popsicles out.

Tips:
• Use 100% fruit juices or purees without added sugars.
• You can mix and match different fruit flavors to create variety.
• For a creamier texture, you can substitute 1/4 cup of the water with unsweetened almond milk or Greek yogurt.
• Adjust the amount of gelatin to achieve your desired firmness.
• Store the popsicles in the freezer for up to 2•3 months.

These sugar•free popsicles can be a refreshing and hydrating option as part of your gastric bypass meal prep. They provide a sweet treat without the added sugars that can be difficult to tolerate after surgery. As always, consult with your healthcare team for any specific dietary recommendations.

10. Protein Shakes (low•sugar, high•protein)

Ingredients:

- 1/2 cup unsweetened almond milk
- 1/4 cup plain Greek yogurt
- 1 scoop chocolate protein powder
- 1 tbsp natural peanut butter
- 1 tsp unsweetened cocoa powder
- 1/2 tsp vanilla extract
- 1•2 ice cubes (optional)

Instructions:

1. Add all the ingredients to a blender.

2. Blend on high speed until smooth and creamy.

3. Taste and adjust any ingredients to your preference.

4. Pour into a small cup or container.

Tips for Gastric Bypass:

• Use smaller portions • this recipe makes a 6•8 oz serving, which is appropriate for post•op gastric bypass.

• Focus on protein and healthy fats • the protein powder, Greek yogurt, and peanut butter provide important nutrients.

• Avoid added sugars • use unsweetened ingredients.

• Blend well to make it easy to digest.

• Sip slowly to avoid dumping syndrome.

This shake provides a satisfying chocolate•peanut butter flavor with a boost of protein, all in a portion size suitable for gastric bypass patients. Adjust the ingredients as needed to meet your personal nutritional goals.

11. Low•fat Milk

Ingredients:

- 1/2 cup low•fat milk
- 1/4 cup plain Greek yogurt
- 1 scoop chocolate protein powder
- 1 tbsp natural peanut butter
- 1 tsp unsweetened cocoa powder
- 1/2 tsp vanilla extract
- 1•2 ice cubes (optional)

Instructions:

1. Add all the ingredients to a blender.

2. Blend on high speed until smooth and creamy.

3. Taste and adjust any ingredients to your preference.

4. Pour into a small cup or container.

Tips for Gastric Bypass:

• Use low•fat milk instead of higher fat dairy to reduce calorie and fat content.

• Stick to a 6•8 oz serving size to avoid dumping syndrome.

• The protein powder, Greek yogurt, and peanut butter provide important nutrients without too much fat or sugar.

• Blend well to make it easy to digest.

• Sip slowly to avoid discomfort.

This shake provides a satisfying chocolate•peanut butter flavor with a boost of protein, all in a portion size suitable for gastric bypass patients. The low•fat milk makes it a bit lighter than using full•fat dairy. Adjust the ingredients as needed to meet your personal nutritional goals.

12. Almond Milk (unsweetened)

Ingredients:

- 1/2 cup unsweetened almond milk
- 1/4 cup plain Greek yogurt
- 1 scoop chocolate protein powder
- 1 tbsp natural peanut butter
- 1 tsp unsweetened cocoa powder
- 1/2 tsp vanilla extract
- 1•2 ice cubes (optional)

Instructions:

1. Add all the ingredients to a blender.

2. Blend on high speed until smooth and creamy.

3. Taste and adjust any ingredients to your preference.

4. Pour into a small cup or container.

Tips for Gastric Bypass:

- Use unsweetened almond milk to keep the carb and calorie content low.

- Stick to a 6•8 oz serving size to avoid dumping syndrome.

- The protein powder, Greek yogurt, and peanut butter provide important nutrients without too much fat or sugar.

- Blend well to make it easy to digest.

- Sip slowly to avoid discomfort.

This shake provides a satisfying chocolate•peanut butter flavor with a boost of protein, all in a portion size suitable for gastric bypass patients. The unsweetened almond milk makes it a lighter, lower•calorie option compared to dairy milk. Adjust the ingredients as needed to meet your personal nutritional goals.

13. Soy Milk (unsweetened)

Ingredients:

- 1/2 cup unsweetened soy milk
- 1/4 cup plain Greek yogurt
- 1 scoop chocolate protein powder
- 1 tbsp natural peanut butter
- 1 tsp unsweetened cocoa powder
- 1/2 tsp vanilla extract
- 1•2 ice cubes (optional)

Instructions:

1. Add all the ingredients to a blender.

2. Blend on high speed until smooth and creamy.

3. Taste and adjust any ingredients to your preference.

4. Pour into a small cup or container.

Tips for Gastric Bypass:

- Use unsweetened soy milk to keep the carb and calorie content low.

- Stick to a 6•8 oz serving size to avoid dumping syndrome.

- The protein powder, Greek yogurt, and peanut butter provide important nutrients without too much fat or sugar.

- Blend well to make it easy to digest.

- Sip slowly to avoid discomfort.

This shake provides a satisfying chocolate•peanut butter flavor with a boost of protein, all in a portion size suitable for gastric bypass patients. The unsweetened soy milk makes it a lighter, lower•calorie option compared to dairy milk. Soy milk is also a good source of plant•based protein. Adjust the ingredients as needed to meet your personal nutritional goals.

14. Strained Cream Soups (low•fat)

Ingredients:

• 1/4 cup low•fat strained cream soup (such as cream of mushroom or cream of chicken)
• 1/4 cup unsweetened almond milk
• 1 scoop chocolate protein powder
• 1 tbsp natural peanut butter
• 1 tsp unsweetened cocoa powder
• 1/2 tsp vanilla extract
• 1•2 ice cubes (optional)

Instructions:

1. Add all the ingredients to a blender.

2. Blend on high speed until smooth and creamy.

3. Taste and adjust any ingredients to your preference.

4. Pour into a small cup or container.

Tips for Gastric Bypass:

• Use a low•fat strained cream soup to add creaminess without too much fat.

• Stick to a 6•8 oz serving size to avoid dumping syndrome.

• The protein powder and peanut butter provide important nutrients.

• Blend well to make it easy to digest.

• Sip slowly to avoid discomfort.

This shake provides a creamy, chocolate•peanut butter flavor with a boost of protein, all in a portion size suitable for gastric bypass patients. The low•fat strained cream soup adds a smooth texture without too many calories or fat. Adjust the ingredients as needed to meet your personal nutritional goals.

Note that the use of strained cream soups in this recipe is a bit unconventional, so you may want to experiment to find the right balance of flavors and textures that work best for you.

15. Greek Yogurt (plain, non•fat)

Ingredients:

- 1/2 cup non•fat plain Greek yogurt
- 1/4 cup unsweetened almond milk
- 1 scoop chocolate protein powder
- 1 tbsp natural peanut butter
- 1 tsp unsweetened cocoa powder
- 1/2 tsp vanilla extract
- 1•2 ice cubes (optional)

Instructions:

1. Add all the ingredients to a blender.

2. Blend on high speed until smooth and creamy.

3. Taste and adjust any ingredients to your preference.

4. Pour into a small cup or container.

Tips for Gastric Bypass:

- Use non•fat plain Greek yogurt to provide protein and creaminess without excess fat.

- Stick to a 6•8 oz serving size to avoid dumping syndrome.

- The protein powder and peanut butter provide additional protein and healthy fats.

- Blend well to make it easy to digest.

- Sip slowly to avoid discomfort.

This shake provides a rich, chocolate•peanut butter flavor with a boost of protein from the Greek yogurt and protein powder. The non•fat Greek yogurt keeps the calorie and fat content low, making it a great option for gastric bypass patients. Adjust the ingredients as needed to meet your personal nutritional goals.

16. Cottage Cheese (blended)

Ingredients:

- 1/4 cup low•fat cottage cheese, blended until smooth
- 1/4 cup unsweetened almond milk
- 1 scoop chocolate protein powder
- 1 tbsp natural peanut butter
- 1 tsp unsweetened cocoa powder
- 1/2 tsp vanilla extract
- 1•2 ice cubes (optional)

Instructions:

1. Add the blended cottage cheese to a blender.

2. Add the remaining ingredients and blend on high speed until smooth and creamy.

3. Taste and adjust any ingredients to your preference.

4. Pour into a small cup or container.

Tips for Gastric Bypass:

- Using blended cottage cheese provides protein and a creamy texture without excess fat.

- Stick to a 6•8 oz serving size to avoid dumping syndrome.

- The protein powder and peanut butter add additional protein and healthy fats.

- Blend well to make it easy to digest.

- Sip slowly to avoid discomfort.

This shake provides a rich, chocolate•peanut butter flavor with a boost of protein from the cottage cheese and protein powder. The low•fat cottage cheese keeps the calorie and fat content low, making it a great option for gastric bypass patients. Adjust the ingredients as needed to meet your personal nutritional goals.

17. Smoothies (fruit, protein powder, unsweetened)

Ingredients:

- 1/2 cup frozen banana slices
- 1/4 cup unsweetened almond milk
- 1 scoop chocolate protein powder
- 1 tbsp natural peanut butter
- 1 tsp unsweetened cocoa powder
- 1/2 tsp vanilla extract

Instructions:

1. Add all the ingredients to a blender.

2. Blend on high speed until smooth and creamy.

3. Taste and adjust any ingredients to your preference.

4. Pour into a small cup or container.

Tips for Gastric Bypass:

- Use frozen banana for natural sweetness and creaminess without added sugar.

- Stick to a 6•8 oz serving size to avoid dumping syndrome.

- The protein powder and peanut butter provide important nutrients.

- Blend well to make it easy to digest.

- Sip slowly to avoid discomfort.

This smoothie provides a delicious chocolate•peanut butter flavor with a boost of protein and nutrients from the fruit, protein powder, and peanut butter. The unsweetened almond milk and lack of added sugars make it a great option for gastric bypass patients. Adjust the ingredients as needed to meet your personal nutritional goals.

18. Pudding (sugar•free)

Ingredients:

- 1/4 cup sugar•free chocolate pudding mix
- 1/2 cup unsweetened almond milk
- 1 tbsp natural peanut butter
- 1 scoop chocolate protein powder
- 1/2 tsp vanilla extract

Instructions:

1. In a small bowl, whisk together the sugar•free chocolate pudding mix and almond milk until smooth and thickened.

2. Stir in the peanut butter, chocolate protein powder, and vanilla extract until well combined.

3. Taste and adjust any ingredients to your preference.

4. Transfer the pudding to a small container.

Tips for Gastric Bypass:

- Use a sugar•free pudding mix to keep the carb and calorie content low.

- Stick to a 4•6 oz serving size to avoid dumping syndrome.

- The protein powder and peanut butter provide important nutrients.

- The thick, creamy texture of the pudding is easy to digest.

- Eat slowly to avoid discomfort.

This sugar•free chocolate peanut butter pudding provides a satisfying dessert•like treat with a boost of protein. The combination of the sugar•free pudding, protein powder, and peanut butter makes it a great option for gastric bypass patients. Adjust the ingredients as needed to meet your personal nutritional goals.

19. Protein Water

Ingredients:

- 1 cup water
- 1 scoop chocolate protein powder
- 1 tbsp natural peanut butter
- 1 tsp unsweetened cocoa powder
- 1/2 tsp vanilla extract
- Ice cubes (optional)

Instructions:

1. In a shaker bottle or blender, combine the water, protein powder, peanut butter, cocoa powder, and vanilla extract.

2. Shake or blend until the ingredients are fully incorporated and the mixture is smooth.

3. Add ice cubes if desired.

4. Pour into a small cup or container.

Tips for Gastric Bypass:

- Protein water provides hydration and protein without the thickness of a traditional shake.

- Stick to a 6•8 oz serving size to avoid dumping syndrome.

- The protein powder and peanut butter provide important nutrients.

- Sip slowly to avoid discomfort.

- Adjust the amount of peanut butter or cocoa powder to suit your taste preferences.

This chocolate peanut butter protein water is a refreshing and easy•to•digest option for gastric bypass patients. The water•based formula is lighter than a traditional shake, while still providing a boost of protein and flavor. Adjust the ingredients as needed to meet your personal nutritional goals.

20. Blended Soups (no chunks)

Ingredients:

- 1/2 cup low•fat cream of mushroom or cream of chicken soup, blended until smooth
- 1/4 cup unsweetened almond milk
- 1 scoop chocolate protein powder
- 1 tbsp natural peanut butter
- 1 tsp unsweetened cocoa powder
- 1/2 tsp vanilla extract

Instructions:

1. In a small saucepan, heat the blended soup over medium heat, stirring occasionally, until warmed through.

2. Remove from heat and transfer the soup to a blender.

3. Add the almond milk, protein powder, peanut butter, cocoa powder, and vanilla extract.

4. Blend on high speed until smooth and well combined.

5. Taste and adjust any ingredients to your preference.

6. Pour into a small bowl or container.

Tips for Gastric Bypass:

- Using a blended, chunky•free soup provides a creamy texture without excess fat or fiber.

- Stick to a 6•8 oz serving size to avoid dumping syndrome.

- The protein powder and peanut butter add important nutrients.

- Sip or eat slowly to avoid discomfort.

- Adjust the amount of soup, milk, or peanut butter to achieve your desired consistency.

This chocolate peanut butter protein soup provides a savory, yet sweet and creamy option for gastric bypass patients. The blended soup base makes it easy to digest, while the protein and healthy fats from the peanut butter help keep you feeling full. Adjust the ingredients as needed to meet your personal nutritional goals.

21. Strained Vegetable Juice

Ingredients:

- 1/2 cup strained vegetable juice (such as carrot, tomato, or V8)
- 1/4 cup unsweetened almond milk
- 1 scoop chocolate protein powder
- 1 tbsp natural peanut butter
- 1 tsp unsweetened cocoa powder
- 1/2 tsp vanilla extract

Instructions:

1. Add all the ingredients to a blender.

2. Blend on high speed until smooth and well combined.

3. Taste and adjust any ingredients to your preference.

4. Pour into a small cup or container.

Tips for Gastric Bypass:

- Use a strained vegetable juice to provide nutrients without excess fiber.

- Stick to a 6•8 oz serving size to avoid dumping syndrome.

- The protein powder and peanut butter add important nutrients.

- Blend well to make it easy to digest.

- Sip slowly to avoid discomfort.

This chocolate peanut butter protein juice provides a unique flavor combination that delivers important vitamins and minerals from the vegetable juice, along with a boost of protein and healthy fats. The strained juice makes it easy to digest, while the other ingredients help keep you feeling full. Adjust the amounts of each ingredient to suit your personal taste and nutritional needs.

22. Scrambled Eggs (soft, pureed)

Ingredients:

- 2 large eggs, scrambled and pureed until smooth
- 1 tbsp unsweetened almond milk
- 1 scoop chocolate protein powder
- 1 tbsp natural peanut butter
- 1 tsp unsweetened cocoa powder
- 1/4 tsp vanilla extract
- Pinch of salt (optional)

Instructions:

1. In a small bowl, whisk together the pureed scrambled eggs and almond milk until well combined.

2. Stir in the chocolate protein powder, peanut butter, cocoa powder, vanilla extract, and salt (if using).

3. Transfer the mixture to a small saucepan and heat over medium•low, stirring frequently, until warmed through.

4. Taste and adjust any seasonings as needed.

5. Transfer to a small bowl or container.

Tips for Gastric Bypass:

- Puree the scrambled eggs to a smooth, creamy consistency for easy digestion.

- Stick to a 4•6 oz serving size to avoid dumping syndrome.

- The protein powder, peanut butter, and cocoa powder provide important nutrients.

- The soft, pureed texture is gentle on the stomach.

- Eat slowly to avoid discomfort.

This chocolate peanut butter protein scrambled egg provides a savory and nutrient•dense option for gastric bypass patients. The pureed texture makes it easy to digest, while the added protein and healthy fats help keep you feeling full. Adjust the ingredients as needed to meet your personal nutritional goals.

23. Mashed Avocado

Ingredients:

- 1/2 ripe avocado, mashed
- 1 tbsp unsweetened almond milk
- 1 scoop chocolate protein powder
- 1 tbsp natural peanut butter
- 1 tsp unsweetened cocoa powder
- 1/2 tsp vanilla extract
- Pinch of salt (optional)

Instructions:

1. In a small bowl, mash the avocado until smooth and creamy.

2. Add the almond milk, protein powder, peanut butter, cocoa powder, vanilla extract, and salt (if using).

3. Stir all the ingredients together until well combined and the mixture is smooth.

4. Taste and adjust any seasonings as needed.

5. Transfer the mashed avocado mixture to a small bowl or container.

Tips for Gastric Bypass:

- Mashed avocado provides healthy fats and a creamy texture.

- Stick to a 4•6 oz serving size to avoid dumping syndrome.

- The protein powder and peanut butter add important nutrients.

- The smooth, soft texture is gentle on the stomach.

- Eat slowly to avoid discomfort.

This chocolate peanut butter protein mashed avocado provides a nutrient•dense and satisfying option for gastric bypass patients. The healthy fats from the avocado, combined with the protein and flavor from the other ingredients, make it a great choice. Adjust the amounts as needed to meet your personal nutritional goals.

24. Refried Beans (fat•free)

Ingredients:

• 1/2 cup fat•free refried beans
• 1 tbsp unsweetened almond milk
• 1 scoop chocolate protein powder
• 1 tbsp natural peanut butter
• 1 tsp unsweetened cocoa powder
• 1/2 tsp ground cinnamon (optional)
• Pinch of salt (optional)

Instructions:

1. In a small bowl, combine the refried beans and almond milk. Stir until well blended and smooth.

2. Add the chocolate protein powder, peanut butter, cocoa powder, cinnamon (if using), and salt (if using). Mix until fully incorporated.

3. Taste and adjust any seasonings as needed.

4. Transfer the bean dip to a small bowl or container.

Tips for Gastric Bypass:

• Use fat•free refried beans to keep the calorie and fat content low.

• Stick to a 4•6 oz serving size to avoid dumping syndrome.

• The protein powder and peanut butter add important nutrients.

• The smooth, creamy texture is gentle on the stomach.

• Dip with low•fat crackers or veggie sticks, or use as a spread.

• Eat slowly to avoid discomfort.

This chocolate peanut butter protein refried bean dip provides a savory and nutrient•dense option for gastric bypass patients. The fat•free beans, protein powder, and peanut butter create a satisfying and easy•to•digest snack or meal component. Adjust the ingredients as needed to meet your personal nutritional goals.

25. Hummus

Ingredients:

- 1/2 cup canned chickpeas, rinsed and drained
- 2 tbsp unsweetened almond milk
- 1 scoop chocolate protein powder
- 1 tbsp natural peanut butter
- 1 tsp unsweetened cocoa powder
- 1/2 tsp ground cumin
- 1/4 tsp garlic powder
- Pinch of salt (optional)

Instructions:

1. In a food processor or high•powered blender, combine the chickpeas, almond milk, protein powder, peanut butter, cocoa powder, cumin, garlic powder, and salt (if using).

2. Blend or process until the mixture is smooth and creamy, scraping down the sides as needed.

3. Taste and adjust any seasonings to your preference.

4. Transfer the chocolate peanut butter protein hummus to a small bowl or container.

Tips for Gastric Bypass:

- Chickpeas provide fiber and protein without excess fat.

- Stick to a 2•4 tbsp serving size to avoid dumping syndrome.

- The protein powder and peanut butter add important nutrients.

- The smooth, creamy texture is gentle on the stomach.

- Dip with low•fat crackers or veggie sticks.

- Eat slowly to avoid discomfort.

This chocolate peanut butter protein hummus provides a unique and nutrient•dense option for gastric bypass patients. The combination of chickpeas, protein powder, and peanut butter creates a satisfying and easy•to•digest snack or meal component. Adjust the ingredients as needed to meet your personal nutritional goals.

26. Pureed Chicken Salad

Ingredients:

- 1/2 cup cooked, shredded chicken breast
- 2 tbsp plain, non•fat Greek yogurt
- 1 tbsp unsweetened almond milk
- 1 scoop chocolate protein powder
- 1 tbsp natural peanut butter
- 1 tsp unsweetened cocoa powder
- 1/4 tsp ground cumin
- Pinch of salt and pepper (optional)

Instructions:

1. In a food processor or high•powered blender, combine the shredded chicken, Greek yogurt, almond milk, protein powder, peanut butter, cocoa powder, cumin, and salt and pepper (if using).

2. Blend or process until the mixture is smooth and creamy, scraping down the sides as needed.

3. Taste and adjust any seasonings to your preference.

4. Transfer the pureed chicken salad to a small bowl or container.

Tips for Gastric Bypass:

- Pureed chicken provides protein without excess fat or fiber.

- Stick to a 2•4 tbsp serving size to avoid dumping syndrome.

- The protein powder and peanut butter add important nutrients.

- The smooth, creamy texture is gentle on the stomach.

- Serve with low•fat crackers or veggie sticks.

- Eat slowly to avoid discomfort.

This chocolate peanut butter protein pureed chicken salad provides a unique and nutrient•dense option for gastric bypass patients. The combination of chicken, protein powder, and peanut butter creates a satisfying and easy•to•digest snack or meal component. Adjust the ingredients as needed to meet your personal nutritional goals.

27. Pureed Tuna Salad

Ingredients:

- 1/2 cup canned tuna, drained
- 2 tbsp plain, non•fat Greek yogurt
- 1 tbsp unsweetened almond milk
- 1 scoop chocolate protein powder
- 1 tbsp natural peanut butter
- 1 tsp unsweetened cocoa powder
- 1/4 tsp ground cumin
- Pinch of salt and pepper (optional)

Instructions:

1. In a food processor or high•powered blender, combine the drained tuna, Greek yogurt, almond milk, protein powder, peanut butter, cocoa powder, cumin, and salt and pepper (if using).

2. Blend or process until the mixture is smooth and creamy, scraping down the sides as needed.

3. Taste and adjust any seasonings to your preference.

4. Transfer the pureed tuna salad to a small bowl or container.

Tips for Gastric Bypass:

- Pureed tuna provides protein without excess fat or fiber.

- Stick to a 2•4 tbsp serving size to avoid dumping syndrome.

- The protein powder and peanut butter add important nutrients.

- The smooth, creamy texture is gentle on the stomach.

- Serve with low•fat crackers or veggie sticks.

- Eat slowly to avoid discomfort.

This chocolate peanut butter protein pureed tuna salad provides a unique and nutrient•dense option for gastric bypass patients. The combination of tuna, protein powder, and peanut butter creates a satisfying and easy•to•digest snack or meal component. Adjust the ingredients as needed to meet your personal nutritional goals.

28. Pureed Salmon Salad

Ingredients:

- 1/2 cup canned salmon, drained and flaked
- 2 tbsp plain, non•fat Greek yogurt
- 1 tbsp unsweetened almond milk
- 1 scoop chocolate protein powder
- 1 tbsp natural peanut butter
- 1 tsp unsweetened cocoa powder
- 1/4 tsp ground dill (optional)
- Pinch of salt and pepper (optional)

Instructions:

1. In a food processor or high•powered blender, combine the flaked salmon, Greek yogurt, almond milk, protein powder, peanut butter, cocoa powder, dill (if using), and salt and pepper (if using).

2. Blend or process until the mixture is smooth and creamy, scraping down the sides as needed.

3. Taste and adjust any seasonings to your preference.

4. Transfer the pureed salmon salad to a small bowl or container.

Tips for Gastric Bypass:

- Pureed salmon provides protein and healthy omega•3 fatty acids without excess fat or fiber.

- Stick to a 2•4 tbsp serving size to avoid dumping syndrome.

- The protein powder and peanut butter add important nutrients.

- The smooth, creamy texture is gentle on the stomach.

- Serve with low•fat crackers or veggie sticks.

- Eat slowly to avoid discomfort.

This chocolate peanut butter protein pureed salmon salad provides a unique and nutrient•dense option for gastric bypass patients. The combination of salmon, protein powder, and peanut butter creates a satisfying and easy•to•digest snack or meal component. Adjust the ingredients as needed to meet your personal nutritional goals.

29. Blended Cottage Cheese (with fruits)

Ingredients:

- 1/2 cup low•fat cottage cheese, blended until smooth
- 1/4 cup unsweetened almond milk
- 1 scoop chocolate protein powder
- 1 tbsp natural peanut butter
- 1/2 cup frozen mixed berries (such as raspberries, blueberries, and strawberries)
- 1 tsp unsweetened cocoa powder

Instructions:

1. In a blender, combine the blended cottage cheese, almond milk, protein powder, and peanut butter. Blend until smooth and creamy.

2. Add the frozen mixed berries and cocoa powder. Blend again until the fruit is fully incorporated and the mixture is well combined.

3. Taste and adjust any ingredients to your preference.

4. Transfer the blended cottage cheese and fruit mixture to a small bowl or container.

Tips for Gastric Bypass:

- The blended cottage cheese provides protein and a creamy texture.

- The frozen fruit adds natural sweetness and nutrients without excess sugar.

- Stick to a 4•6 oz serving size to avoid dumping syndrome.

- The protein powder and peanut butter contribute important nutrients.

- The smooth, blended consistency is gentle on the stomach.

- Eat slowly to avoid discomfort.

This chocolate peanut butter protein blended cottage cheese with fruit provides a nutrient•dense and satisfying option for gastric bypass patients. The combination of protein, healthy fats, and natural sweetness from the fruit makes it a great choice. Adjust the ingredients as needed to meet your personal nutritional goals.

30. Pureed Vegetables (carrots, peas, etc.)

Ingredients:

- 1/2 cup pureed cooked vegetables (such as carrots, peas, or a vegetable blend)
- 1/4 cup unsweetened almond milk
- 1 scoop chocolate protein powder
- 1 tbsp natural peanut butter
- 1 tsp unsweetened cocoa powder
- 1/4 tsp ground cinnamon (optional)
- Pinch of salt (optional)

Instructions:

1. In a blender or food processor, combine the pureed vegetables, almond milk, protein powder, peanut butter, cocoa powder, cinnamon (if using), and salt (if using).

2. Blend or process until the mixture is smooth and creamy, scraping down the sides as needed.

3. Taste and adjust any seasonings to your preference.

4. Transfer the pureed vegetable blend to a small bowl or container.

Tips for Gastric Bypass:

- Using a pureed vegetable blend provides nutrients without excess fiber.

- Stick to a 4•6 oz serving size to avoid dumping syndrome.

- The protein powder and peanut butter add important nutrients.

- The smooth, creamy texture is gentle on the stomach.

- The cinnamon (optional) can add a subtle warmth and flavor.

- Eat slowly to avoid discomfort.

This chocolate peanut butter protein pureed vegetable blend provides a nutrient•dense and easy•to•digest option for gastric bypass patients. The combination of pureed vegetables, protein powder, and peanut butter creates a satisfying and versatile snack or meal component. Adjust the ingredients as needed to meet your personal nutritional goals.

31. Pureed Fruits (applesauce, banana)

Ingredients:

- 1/2 cup pureed fruit (such as applesauce or mashed banana)
- 1/4 cup unsweetened almond milk
- 1 scoop chocolate protein powder
- 1 tbsp natural peanut butter
- 1 tsp unsweetened cocoa powder
- 1/2 tsp vanilla extract
- Pinch of cinnamon (optional)

Instructions:

1. In a blender or food processor, combine the pureed fruit, almond milk, protein powder, peanut butter, cocoa powder, vanilla extract, and cinnamon (if using).

2. Blend or process until the mixture is smooth and creamy, scraping down the sides as needed.
3. Taste and adjust any ingredients to your preference.

4. Transfer the pureed fruit blend to a small bowl or container.

Tips for Gastric Bypass:

- Using pureed fruits provides natural sweetness and nutrients without excess fiber.

- Stick to a 4•6 oz serving size to avoid dumping syndrome.

- The protein powder and peanut butter add important nutrients.

- The smooth, creamy texture is gentle on the stomach.

- The cinnamon (optional) can add a subtle warmth and flavor.

- Eat slowly to avoid discomfort.

This chocolate peanut butter protein pureed fruit blend provides a nutrient•dense and easy•to•digest option for gastric bypass patients. The combination of pureed fruit, protein powder, and peanut butter creates a satisfying and versatile snack or meal component. Adjust the ingredients as needed to meet your personal nutritional goals.

32. Tofu (silken, blended)

Ingredients:

• 1/2 cup silken tofu, blended until smooth
• 1/4 cup unsweetened almond milk
• 1 scoop chocolate protein powder
• 1 tbsp natural peanut butter
• 1 tsp unsweetened cocoa powder
• 1/2 tsp vanilla extract
• Pinch of salt (optional)

Instructions:

1. In a blender or food processor, combine the blended silken tofu, almond milk, protein powder, peanut butter, cocoa powder, vanilla extract, and salt (if using).

2. Blend or process until the mixture is smooth and creamy, scraping down the sides as needed.

3. Taste and adjust any ingredients to your preference.

4. Transfer the silken tofu blend to a small bowl or container.

Tips for Gastric Bypass:

• Silken tofu provides protein and a creamy texture without excess fat.

• Stick to a 4•6 oz serving size to avoid dumping syndrome.

• The protein powder and peanut butter add important nutrients.

• The smooth, blended consistency is gentle on the stomach.

• The vanilla and cocoa powder provide flavor without added sugar.

• Eat slowly to avoid discomfort.

This chocolate peanut butter protein silken tofu blend provides a nutrient•dense and easy•to•digest option for gastric bypass patients. The combination of blended tofu, protein powder, and peanut butter creates a satisfying and versatile snack or meal component. Adjust the ingredients as needed to meet your personal nutritional goals.

33. Greek Yogurt Smoothies

Ingredients:

- 1/2 cup plain, non•fat Greek yogurt
- 1/4 cup unsweetened almond milk
- 1 scoop chocolate protein powder
- 1 tbsp natural peanut butter
- 1 tsp unsweetened cocoa powder
- 1/2 tsp vanilla extract
- 1•2 ice cubes (optional)

Instructions:

1. Add all the ingredients to a blender.

2. Blend on high speed until smooth and creamy.

3. Taste and adjust any ingredients to your preference.

4. Pour into a small cup or container.

Tips for Gastric Bypass:

- Greek yogurt provides protein and a creamy texture.

- Stick to a 6•8 oz serving size to avoid dumping syndrome.

- The protein powder and peanut butter add important nutrients.

- The smooth, blended consistency is gentle on the stomach.

- The cocoa powder and vanilla extract provide flavor without added sugar.

- Sip slowly to avoid discomfort.

This chocolate peanut butter protein Greek yogurt smoothie provides a nutrient•dense and satisfying option for gastric bypass patients. The combination of Greek yogurt, protein powder, and peanut butter creates a creamy, flavorful smoothie that is easy to digest. Adjust the ingredients as needed to meet your personal nutritional goals.

34. Lentil Soup (pureed)

Ingredients:
- 1/2 cup pureed lentil soup
- 1/4 cup unsweetened almond milk
- 1 scoop chocolate protein powder
- 1 tbsp natural peanut butter
- 1 tsp unsweetened cocoa powder
- 1/4 tsp ground cumin
- Pinch of salt and pepper (optional)

Instructions:
1. In a small saucepan, warm the pureed lentil soup over medium heat, stirring occasionally.

2. Once heated through, transfer the soup to a blender.

3. Add the almond milk, protein powder, peanut butter, cocoa powder, cumin, and salt and pepper (if using).

4. Blend on high speed until the mixture is smooth and well combined.

5. Taste and adjust any seasonings to your preference.

6. Pour the pureed lentil soup into a small bowl or container.

Tips for Gastric Bypass:
- Pureed lentil soup provides protein, fiber, and nutrients without excess texture.

- Stick to a 4•6 oz serving size to avoid dumping syndrome.

- The protein powder and peanut butter add important nutrients.

- The smooth, creamy texture is gentle on the stomach.

- The cocoa powder and cumin add flavor without added sugar.

- Eat slowly to avoid discomfort.

This chocolate peanut butter protein pureed lentil soup provides a savory and nutrient•dense option for gastric bypass patients. The combination of the pureed lentil base, protein powder, and peanut butter creates a satisfying and easy•to•digest meal. Adjust the ingredients as needed to meet your personal nutritional goals.

35. Pureed Tofu and Vegetable Soup

Ingredients:

- 1/2 cup pureed tofu and vegetable soup (such as a creamy tomato or butternut squash soup)
- 1/4 cup unsweetened almond milk
- 1 scoop chocolate protein powder
- 1 tbsp natural peanut butter
- 1 tsp unsweetened cocoa powder
- 1/4 tsp ground cinnamon (optional)
- Pinch of salt and pepper (optional)

Instructions:

1. In a small saucepan, warm the pureed tofu and vegetable soup over medium heat, stirring occasionally.

2. Once heated through, transfer the soup to a blender.

3. Add the almond milk, protein powder, peanut butter, cocoa powder, cinnamon (if using), and salt and pepper (if using).

4. Blend on high speed until the mixture is smooth and well combined.

5. Taste and adjust any seasonings to your preference. Pour the pureed soup into a small bowl or container.

Tips for Gastric Bypass:

- Pureed tofu and vegetable soup provides protein, fiber, and nutrients without excess texture.

- Stick to a 4•6 oz serving size to avoid dumping syndrome.

- The protein powder and peanut butter add important nutrients.

- The smooth, creamy texture is gentle on the stomach.

- The cocoa powder and cinnamon (optional) add flavor without added sugar. Eat slowly to avoid discomfort.

This chocolate peanut butter protein pureed tofu and vegetable soup provides a savory and nutrient•dense option for gastric bypass patients. The combination of the pureed soup base, protein powder, and peanut butter creates a satisfying and easy•to•digest meal. Adjust the ingredients as needed to meet your personal nutritional goals.

36. Pureed Sweet Potato

Ingredients:

- 1/2 cup pureed cooked sweet potato
- 1/4 cup unsweetened almond milk
- 1 scoop chocolate protein powder
- 1 tbsp natural peanut butter
- 1 tsp unsweetened cocoa powder
- 1/4 tsp ground cinnamon
- Pinch of salt (optional)

Instructions:

1. In a blender or food processor, combine the pureed sweet potato, almond milk, protein powder, peanut butter, cocoa powder, cinnamon, and salt (if using).

2. Blend or process until the mixture is smooth and creamy, scraping down the sides as needed.

3. Taste and adjust any ingredients to your preference.

4. Transfer the pureed sweet potato to a small bowl or container.

Tips for Gastric Bypass:

- Pureed sweet potato provides fiber, vitamins, and a naturally sweet flavor.

- Stick to a 4•6 oz serving size to avoid dumping syndrome.

- The protein powder and peanut butter add important nutrients.

- The smooth, creamy texture is gentle on the stomach.

- The cinnamon adds warmth and flavor without added sugar.

- Eat slowly to avoid discomfort.

This chocolate peanut butter protein pureed sweet potato provides a nutrient•dense and easy•to•digest option for gastric bypass patients. The combination of the sweet potato, protein powder, and peanut butter creates a satisfying and versatile snack or meal component. Adjust the ingredients as needed to meet your personal nutritional goals.

37. Soft•cooked Eggs

Ingredients:

- 2 large eggs, soft•cooked
- 1 tbsp unsweetened almond milk
- 1 scoop chocolate protein powder
- 1 tbsp natural peanut butter
- 1 tsp unsweetened cocoa powder
- 1/4 tsp vanilla extract
- Pinch of salt and pepper (optional)

Instructions:

1. In a small bowl, gently break the soft•cooked eggs and mash them with a fork until they are broken up but still have a soft, creamy texture.

2. Add the almond milk, protein powder, peanut butter, cocoa powder, vanilla extract, and salt and pepper (if using). Stir until well combined.

3. Taste and adjust any seasonings to your preference.

4. Transfer the chocolate peanut butter protein soft•cooked eggs to a small bowl or container.

Tips for Gastric Bypass:

- Soft•cooked eggs are easy to digest and provide protein.

- Stick to a 2•4 tbsp serving size to avoid dumping syndrome.

- The protein powder and peanut butter add important nutrients.

- The smooth, creamy texture is gentle on the stomach.

- The cocoa powder and vanilla extract provide flavor without added sugar.

- Eat slowly to avoid discomfort.

This chocolate peanut butter protein soft•cooked egg dish provides a savory and nutrient•dense option for gastric bypass patients. The combination of the soft•cooked eggs, protein powder, and peanut butter creates a satisfying and easy•to•digest meal. Adjust the ingredients as needed to meet your personal nutritional goals.

38. Oatmeal (runny consistency)

Ingredients:

- 1/2 cup cooked oatmeal, thinned with extra liquid to a runny consistency
- 1/4 cup unsweetened almond milk
- 1 scoop chocolate protein powder
- 1 tbsp natural peanut butter
- 1 tsp unsweetened cocoa powder
- 1/2 tsp vanilla extract
- Pinch of cinnamon (optional)

Instructions:

1. In a small bowl, combine the runny oatmeal and almond milk. Stir until well blended.

2. Add the chocolate protein powder, peanut butter, cocoa powder, vanilla extract, and cinnamon (if using). Mix until fully incorporated.

3. Taste and adjust any ingredients to your preference.

4. Transfer the chocolate peanut butter protein runny oatmeal to a small bowl or container.

Tips for Gastric Bypass:

- Thinning the oatmeal to a runny consistency makes it easier to digest.

- Stick to a 4•6 oz serving size to avoid dumping syndrome.

- The protein powder and peanut butter add important nutrients.

- The smooth, creamy texture is gentle on the stomach.

- The cocoa powder, vanilla, and cinnamon (optional) provide flavor without added sugar.

- Eat slowly to avoid discomfort.

This chocolate peanut butter protein runny oatmeal provides a warm, comforting, and nutrient•dense option for gastric bypass patients. The combination of the thinned oatmeal, protein powder, and peanut butter creates a satisfying and easy•to•digest meal. Adjust the ingredients as needed to meet your personal nutritional goals.

39. Cream of Wheat

Ingredients:

- 1/2 cup cooked Cream of Wheat, thinned with extra liquid to a smooth, runny consistency
- 1/4 cup unsweetened almond milk
- 1 scoop chocolate protein powder
- 1 tbsp natural peanut butter
- 1 tsp unsweetened cocoa powder
- 1/2 tsp vanilla extract
- Pinch of ground cinnamon (optional)

Instructions:

1. In a small saucepan, combine the thinned Cream of Wheat and almond milk. Heat over medium, stirring frequently, until warmed through.

2. Remove from heat and transfer the mixture to a small bowl.

3. Stir in the chocolate protein powder, peanut butter, cocoa powder, vanilla extract, and cinnamon (if using) until well blended.

4. Taste and adjust any ingredients to your preference.

5. Transfer the chocolate peanut butter protein Cream of Wheat to a small bowl or container.

Tips for Gastric Bypass:

- Thinning the Cream of Wheat to a smooth, runny consistency makes it easier to digest.

- Stick to a 4•6 oz serving size to avoid dumping syndrome.

- The protein powder and peanut butter add important nutrients.

- The smooth, creamy texture is gentle on the stomach.

- The cocoa powder, vanilla, and cinnamon (optional) provide flavor without added sugar. Eat slowly to avoid discomfort.

This chocolate peanut butter protein Cream of Wheat provides a warm, comforting, and nutrient•dense option for gastric bypass patients. The combination of the thinned Cream of Wheat, protein powder, and peanut butter creates a satisfying and easy•to•digest meal. Adjust the ingredients as needed to meet your personal nutritional goals.

40. Soft Fish (tilapia, cod)

Ingredients:

- 1/2 cup cooked, flaked soft fish (such as tilapia or cod)
- 1/4 cup unsweetened almond milk
- 1 scoop chocolate protein powder
- 1 tbsp natural peanut butter
- 1 tsp unsweetened cocoa powder
- 1/4 tsp ground cumin
- Pinch of salt and pepper (optional)

Instructions:

1. In a food processor or blender, combine the cooked, flaked fish, almond milk, protein powder, peanut butter, cocoa powder, cumin, and salt and pepper (if using).

2. Blend or process until the mixture is smooth and creamy, scraping down the sides as needed.

3. Taste and adjust any seasonings to your preference.

4. Transfer the pureed soft fish to a small bowl or container.

Tips for Gastric Bypass:

- Pureed soft fish provides protein and omega•3 fatty acids without excess texture.

- Stick to a 4•6 oz serving size to avoid dumping syndrome.

- The protein powder and peanut butter add important nutrients.

- The smooth, creamy texture is gentle on the stomach.

- The cocoa powder and cumin add flavor without added sugar.

- Eat slowly to avoid discomfort.

This chocolate peanut butter protein pureed soft fish provides a savory and nutrient•dense option for gastric bypass patients. The combination of the pureed fish, protein powder, and peanut butter creates a satisfying and easy•to•digest meal. Adjust the ingredients as needed to meet your personal nutritional goals.

41. Soft Tofu

Ingredients:

- 1/2 cup soft or silken tofu, mashed
- 1/4 cup unsweetened almond milk
- 1 scoop chocolate protein powder
- 1 tbsp natural peanut butter
- 1 tsp unsweetened cocoa powder
- 1/2 tsp vanilla extract
- Pinch of salt (optional)

Instructions:

1. In a small bowl, mash the soft or silken tofu with a fork until it has a smooth, creamy texture.

2. Add the almond milk, protein powder, peanut butter, cocoa powder, vanilla extract, and salt (if using). Stir until well combined.

3. Taste and adjust any ingredients to your preference.

4. Transfer the chocolate peanut butter protein soft tofu to a small bowl or container.

Tips for Gastric Bypass:

- Soft or silken tofu provides protein and a creamy texture without excess fiber.

- Stick to a 4•6 oz serving size to avoid dumping syndrome.

- The protein powder and peanut butter add important nutrients.

- The smooth, soft texture is gentle on the stomach.

- The cocoa powder and vanilla extract provide flavor without added sugar.

- Eat slowly to avoid discomfort.

This chocolate peanut butter protein soft tofu provides a nutrient•dense and easy•to•digest option for gastric bypass patients. The combination of the mashed tofu, protein powder, and peanut butter creates a satisfying and versatile snack or meal component. Adjust the ingredients as needed to meet your personal nutritional goals.

42. Soft Cheese (mozzarella, ricotta)

Ingredients:

• 1/4 cup soft cheese (such as mozzarella or ricotta), softened
• 1/4 cup unsweetened almond milk
• 1 scoop chocolate protein powder
• 1 tbsp natural peanut butter
• 1 tsp unsweetened cocoa powder
• 1/2 tsp vanilla extract
• Pinch of salt (optional)

Instructions:

1. In a small bowl, combine the softened soft cheese and almond milk. Stir until well blended and smooth.

2. Add the chocolate protein powder, peanut butter, cocoa powder, vanilla extract, and salt (if using). Mix until fully incorporated.

3. Taste and adjust any ingredients to your preference.

4. Transfer the chocolate peanut butter protein soft cheese spread to a small bowl or container.

Tips for Gastric Bypass:

• Soft cheeses like mozzarella and ricotta provide protein and a creamy texture.

• Stick to a 2•4 tbsp serving size to avoid dumping syndrome.

• The protein powder and peanut butter add important nutrients.

• The smooth, soft texture is gentle on the stomach.

• The cocoa powder and vanilla extract provide flavor without added sugar.

• Serve with low•fat crackers or veggie sticks.

• Eat slowly to avoid discomfort.

This chocolate peanut butter protein soft cheese spread provides a nutrient•dense and easy•to•digest option for gastric bypass patients. The combination of the soft cheese, protein powder, and peanut butter creates a satisfying and versatile snack or meal component. Adjust the ingredients as needed to meet your personal nutritional goals.

43. Canned Fruit (in water, no sugar added)

Ingredients:

- 1/2 cup canned fruit (such as peaches, pears, or mandarin oranges), drained and pureed
- 1/4 cup unsweetened almond milk
- 1 scoop chocolate protein powder
- 1 tbsp natural peanut butter
- 1 tsp unsweetened cocoa powder
- 1/2 tsp vanilla extract

Instructions:

1. In a blender or food processor, combine the pureed canned fruit, almond milk, protein powder, peanut butter, cocoa powder, and vanilla extract.

2. Blend or process until the mixture is smooth and well combined.

3. Taste and adjust any ingredients to your preference.

4. Transfer the chocolate peanut butter protein canned fruit puree to a small bowl or container.

Tips for Gastric Bypass:

- Use canned fruit packed in water or its own juice, without added sugar.

- Stick to a 4•6 oz serving size to avoid dumping syndrome.

- The protein powder and peanut butter add important nutrients

- The smooth, creamy texture is gentle on the stomach.

- The cocoa powder and vanilla extract provide flavor without added sugar.

- Eat slowly to avoid discomfort.

This chocolate peanut butter protein canned fruit puree provides a nutrient•dense and easy•to•digest option for gastric bypass patients. The combination of the pureed fruit, protein powder, and peanut butter creates a satisfying and versatile snack or meal component. Adjust the ingredients as needed to meet your personal nutritional goals.

44. Soft•cooked Vegetables

Ingredients:

• 1 lb mixed vegetables (such as carrots, broccoli, cauliflower, zucchini, etc.), chopped into small pieces
• 1/4 cup low•sodium broth or water
• 1 tbsp butter or olive oil
• Salt and pepper to taste

Instructions:

1. In a medium saucepan, combine the chopped vegetables and broth/water. Bring to a boil over high heat.

2. Once boiling, reduce heat to low, cover the pan, and let the vegetables steam for 10•15 minutes, until very soft and tender. Check occasionally and add more liquid if needed to prevent sticking or burning.

3. Drain any excess liquid from the pan. Add the butter or olive oil and gently toss to coat the vegetables.

4. Season with a small amount of salt and pepper to taste.

5. Serve the soft•cooked vegetables warm. They can be mashed or puréed further if needed for easier digestion after gastric bypass.

Tips:
• Choose a variety of nutrient•dense vegetables.

• Cook the vegetables until they are very soft and tender.

• Avoid overcooking, which can make the vegetables mushy.

• Portion into individual servings for easy meal prep.

This simple soft•cooked vegetable dish provides vitamins, minerals, and fiber in an easy•to•digest form, making it a great option for gastric bypass patients. Adjust cooking time as needed to achieve the desired texture.

45. Mashed Potatoes (without butter)

Ingredients:

- 2 lbs russet or Yukon Gold potatoes, peeled and cut into 1•inch cubes
- 1/2 cup low•fat milk or unsweetened almond milk
- 1/4 cup low•sodium chicken or vegetable broth
- 1/2 tsp garlic powder
- 1/4 tsp onion powder
- Salt and pepper to taste

Instructions:

1. Place the cubed potatoes in a large pot and cover with cold water by 1 inch. Bring to a boil over high heat.

2. Once boiling, reduce heat to medium•low and simmer for 15•20 minutes, until the potatoes are very soft when pierced with a fork.

3. Drain the potatoes well in a colander. Return the potatoes to the pot.

4. Add the milk, broth, garlic powder, and onion powder. Mash the potatoes with a potato masher or hand mixer until smooth and creamy.

5. Season with a small amount of salt and pepper to taste.

6. Serve the mashed potatoes warm.

Tips:
- Use a ricer or food mill for an extra smooth texture.

- For a creamier consistency, add a bit more milk or broth.

- Adjust seasoning as needed.

- Portion into individual servings for easy meal prep.

This simple mashed potato recipe omits butter but still provides a creamy, flavorful side dish that is easy to digest after gastric bypass surgery. The milk and broth help keep the potatoes moist and smooth.

46. Ground Turkey

Ingredients:

• 1 lb ground turkey (93% lean or higher)
• 1 tsp olive oil
• 1/2 onion, finely diced
• 2 cloves garlic, minced
• 1 tsp dried oregano
• 1/2 tsp dried basil
• 1/4 tsp red pepper flakes (optional)
• Salt and pepper to taste

Instructions:

1. In a large skillet or non•stick pan, heat the olive oil over medium heat.

2. Add the diced onion and sauté for 2•3 minutes until translucent.

3. Add the minced garlic and sauté for 1 minute until fragrant.

4. Crumble the ground turkey into the pan and cook, breaking it up with a wooden spoon, until no longer pink, about 5•7 minutes.

5. Stir in the dried oregano, basil, and red pepper flakes (if using). Season with a small amount of salt and pepper to taste.

6. Continue cooking for 2•3 minutes, stirring occasionally, until the turkey is cooked through.

7. Remove from heat and let cool slightly before portioning out.

Tips:
• Use 93% lean or higher ground turkey to minimize fat content.

• Adjust seasoning to your taste preferences.

• Portion into individual servings for easy meal prep.

• Ground turkey can be used in a variety of dishes like tacos, casseroles, soups, etc.

This simple ground turkey recipe provides a lean protein source that is easy to incorporate into meals after gastric bypass surgery. It can be a versatile base for many different dishes.

47. Ground Chicken

Ingredients:

- 1 lb ground chicken (93% lean or higher)
- 1 tsp olive oil
- 1/2 onion, finely diced
- 2 cloves garlic, minced
- 1 tsp dried parsley
- 1/2 tsp dried thyme
- 1/4 tsp ground black pepper
- 1/4 tsp salt (or to taste)

Instructions:

1. In a large skillet or non•stick pan, heat the olive oil over medium heat.

2. Add the diced onion and sauté for 2•3 minutes until translucent.

3. Add the minced garlic and sauté for 1 minute until fragrant.

4. Crumble the ground chicken into the pan and cook, breaking it up with a wooden spoon, until no longer pink, about 5•7 minutes.

5. Stir in the dried parsley, thyme, black pepper, and salt.

6. Continue cooking for 2•3 minutes, stirring occasionally, until the chicken is cooked through.

7. Remove from heat and let cool slightly before portioning out.

Tips:
- Use 93% lean or higher ground chicken to minimize fat content.

- Adjust seasoning to your taste preferences.

- Portion into individual servings for easy meal prep.

- Ground chicken can be used in a variety of dishes like burgers, meatballs, casseroles, soups, etc.

This simple ground chicken recipe provides a lean protein source that is easy to incorporate into meals after gastric bypass surgery. It can be a versatile base for many different dishes.

48. Ground Beef (extra lean)

Ingredients:

- 1 lb extra lean ground beef (96% lean or higher)
- 1 tsp olive oil
- 1/2 onion, finely diced
- 2 cloves garlic, minced
- 1 tsp dried oregano
- 1/2 tsp dried basil
- 1/4 tsp red pepper flakes (optional)
- Salt and pepper to taste

Instructions:

1. In a large skillet or non•stick pan, heat the olive oil over medium heat.

2. Add the diced onion and sauté for 2•3 minutes until translucent.

3. Add the minced garlic and sauté for 1 minute until fragrant.

4. Crumble the extra lean ground beef into the pan and cook, breaking it up with a wooden spoon, until no longer pink, about 5•7 minutes.

5. Stir in the dried oregano, basil, and red pepper flakes (if using). Season with a small amount of salt and pepper to taste.

6. Continue cooking for 2•3 minutes, stirring occasionally, until the beef is cooked through.

7. Remove from heat and let cool slightly before portioning out.

Tips:
- Use 96% lean or higher ground beef to minimize fat content.
- Adjust seasoning to your taste preferences.
- Portion into individual servings for easy meal prep.
- Extra lean ground beef can be used in a variety of dishes like burgers, meatballs, chili, casseroles, etc.

This extra lean ground beef recipe provides a protein•rich option that is low in fat, making it a good choice for meal prep after gastric bypass surgery. The simple seasoning allows the beef to be versatile in many different dishes.

49. Soft Meatballs (turkey, chicken)

Ingredients:

- 1 lb ground turkey or ground chicken (93% lean or higher)
- 1/4 cup low•fat milk
- 1/4 cup breadcrumbs or panko
- 1 egg, lightly beaten
- 2 tbsp finely chopped onion
- 1 clove garlic, minced
- 1 tsp dried parsley
- 1/2 tsp dried oregano
- 1/4 tsp salt
- 1/4 tsp black pepper

Instructions:

1. Preheat oven to 375°F. Line a baking sheet with parchment paper.

2. In a large bowl, combine the ground turkey/chicken, milk, breadcrumbs, egg, onion, garlic, parsley, oregano, salt, and pepper. Mix gently until just combined, being careful not to overmix.

3. Scoop the mixture by heaping tablespoons and roll into small, soft meatballs, about 1•inch in size.

4. Place the meatballs on the prepared baking sheet, spacing them apart.

5. Bake for 18•20 minutes, until the meatballs are cooked through and no longer pink in the center.

6. Let the meatballs cool slightly before serving or portioning out.

Tips:
- Use 93% lean or higher ground turkey or chicken to minimize fat content.
- For an extra soft texture, add a bit more milk or breadcrumbs.
- Adjust seasoning to your taste preferences.
- Portion the meatballs into individual servings for easy meal prep.
- Serve the meatballs over mashed potatoes, rice, or with soft•cooked vegetables.

These soft, tender meatballs made with lean ground turkey or chicken provide a protein•rich option that is easy to digest after gastric bypass surgery. The simple seasoning makes them versatile for many different meals.

50. Smooth Nut Butters (peanut, almond)

Ingredients:

Tips for using smooth nut butters:

• Choose natural, unsweetened nut butters without added sugars or oils. Look for just nuts as the sole ingredient.

• Opt for smooth/creamy varieties over crunchy. The smooth texture is easier to digest.

• Start with very small portions, like 1•2 tablespoons at a time. Nut butters are calorie•dense.

• Mix nut butter into other soft, pureed foods like yogurt, oatmeal, or mashed sweet potatoes.

• Use nut butter as a dip for soft, cooked vegetables.

• Drizzle a small amount over cooked proteins like chicken or fish.

• Avoid eating nut butters on their own, as the texture can be difficult to tolerate early on.

Some ideas for incorporating smooth nut butters:

• Peanut butter mixed into Greek yogurt

• Almond butter swirled into mashed sweet potatoes

• Peanut butter drizzled over soft•cooked chicken and broccoli

• Almond butter used as a dip for steamed carrots

Start with very small portions and pay attention to how your body tolerates the nut butters. Adjust amounts as needed. Smooth nut butters can be a nutritious addition to your post•op gastric bypass meal plan.

51. Steamed Cauliflower (mashed)

Ingredients:

- 1 head of cauliflower, cut into florets
- 1/4 cup low•sodium chicken or vegetable broth
- 2 tbsp unsweetened almond milk or low•fat milk
- 1/4 tsp garlic powder
- 1/4 tsp onion powder
- Salt and pepper to taste

Instructions:

1. In a large steamer basket or pot with a steamer insert, bring 1•2 inches of water to a boil over high heat.

2. Add the cauliflower florets to the steamer basket, cover, and steam for 12•15 minutes, until very soft and tender.

3. Carefully transfer the steamed cauliflower to a food processor or blender. Add the broth, milk, garlic powder, and onion powder.

4. Blend or process the cauliflower mixture until smooth and creamy, scraping down the sides as needed.

5. Season with a small amount of salt and pepper to taste.

6. Serve the mashed cauliflower warm.

Tips:
- For a thicker consistency, use less broth/milk.

- For a creamier texture, add a bit more milk.

- Adjust seasoning to your preferences.

- Portion the mashed cauliflower into individual servings for easy meal prep.

This simple steamed and mashed cauliflower dish provides a soft, easy•to•digest vegetable option that can be a great side dish or base for other meals after gastric bypass surgery. The mild flavor and smooth texture make it very versatile.

52. Soft Rice (brown, wild)

Ingredients:

• 1 cup brown rice or wild rice
• 2 cups low•sodium chicken or vegetable broth
• 1/4 tsp salt (optional)

Instructions:

1. In a medium saucepan, combine the rice, broth, and salt (if using).

2. Bring the mixture to a boil over high heat.

3. Once boiling, reduce the heat to low, cover the pan, and simmer for 30•40 minutes, until the rice is very soft and tender.

4. Check the rice periodically and add more broth if needed to prevent sticking or drying out.

5. Once the rice is cooked through, remove from heat and let sit, covered, for 5 minutes.

6. Fluff the rice with a fork before serving or portioning out.

Tips:
• Use low•sodium broth to control salt intake.

• Cook the rice until it is very soft and mushy in texture.

• Adjust cooking time as needed to achieve the desired softness.

• Portion the cooked rice into individual servings for easy meal prep.

This simple method for cooking brown or wild rice results in a soft, easy•to•digest texture that is well•suited for gastric bypass patients. The rice can be a versatile base for other soft, pureed foods or served on its own.

53. Greek Yogurt Parfait (with berries)

Ingredients:

- 1 cup plain, unsweetened Greek yogurt
- 1/2 cup fresh or frozen berries (such as blueberries, raspberries, or blackberries)
- 1•2 tsp honey or maple syrup (optional)

Instructions:

1. In a small bowl or parfait glass, layer half of the Greek yogurt.

2. Top the yogurt with half of the berries.

3. Repeat the layers, ending with the remaining berries on top.

4. If desired, drizzle 1•2 tsp of honey or maple syrup over the top.

5. Serve chilled or at room temperature.

Tips:
- Use plain, unsweetened Greek yogurt for a higher protein content.

- Choose soft, easy•to•digest berries like blueberries or raspberries.

- Start with small portions and adjust the amount of yogurt and berries as needed.

- The honey or maple syrup is optional, as the berries provide natural sweetness.

- Portion the parfait into individual servings for easy meal prep.

This Greek yogurt parfait provides a nutrient•dense, protein•rich breakfast or snack option that is soft and easy to digest after gastric bypass surgery. The combination of creamy yogurt and sweet berries makes it a satisfying and flavorful choice.

54. Protein Pancakes

Ingredients:

• 1/2 cup rolled oats
• 1/2 cup low•fat cottage cheese
• 2 eggs
• 1 scoop (about 25g) vanilla protein powder
• 1 tsp baking powder
• 1/4 tsp cinnamon (optional)
• Nonstick cooking spray

Instructions:

1. In a blender or food processor, blend the rolled oats until they reach a flour•like consistency.

2. Add the cottage cheese, eggs, protein powder, baking powder, and cinnamon (if using). Blend until the batter is smooth and well combined.

3. Heat a nonstick skillet or griddle over medium heat and lightly coat with nonstick cooking spray.

4. Scoop the batter by 1/4 cup portions onto the hot surface, forming small pancakes.

5. Cook for 2•3 minutes per side, until the pancakes are lightly golden brown.

6. Serve the protein pancakes warm, with optional toppings like fresh berries, a drizzle of maple syrup, or a spoonful of Greek yogurt.

Tips:
• Use a vanilla or unflavored protein powder for the best texture.

• Adjust the amount of protein powder to your preference and dietary needs.

• Portion the cooked pancakes into individual servings for easy meal prep.

• Reheat gently before serving.

These protein•packed pancakes provide a nutrient•dense and satisfying breakfast option that is easy to digest after gastric bypass surgery. The combination of oats, cottage cheese, and protein powder makes them a great source of protein, fiber, and complex carbohydrates.

55. Egg White Omelette (with spinach)

Ingredients:

- 4 egg whites
- 1 cup fresh spinach, chopped
- 1 tbsp low•fat milk or unsweetened almond milk
- 1/4 tsp garlic powder
- 1/4 tsp onion powder
- Salt and pepper to taste
- Nonstick cooking spray

Instructions:

1. In a small bowl, whisk together the egg whites, milk, garlic powder, and onion powder until well combined.

2. Spray a nonstick skillet or omelet pan with cooking spray and heat over medium heat.

3. Pour the egg white mixture into the pan and let it cook for 2•3 minutes, until the bottom is set.

4. Sprinkle the chopped spinach over the top of the egg whites.

5. Using a spatula, gently fold the omelet in half and continue cooking for another 2•3 minutes, until the spinach is wilted and the egg is cooked through.

6. Slide the omelet onto a plate and season with a small amount of salt and pepper to taste.

7. Serve the egg white omelet warm.

Tips:
- Use fresh spinach for the best texture and flavor.
- Adjust the amount of spinach to your preference.
- For a creamier texture, add a bit more milk.
- Portion the cooked omelet into individual servings for easy meal prep.
- Reheat gently before serving.

This simple egg white omelet with spinach provides a protein•rich, nutrient•dense meal that is easy to digest after gastric bypass surgery. The soft, smooth texture makes it a great option for post•op meal prep.

56. Cottage Cheese (with pineapple)

Ingredients:

- 1 cup low•fat or non•fat cottage cheese
- 1/2 cup diced fresh or canned pineapple (in its own juice, not syrup)
- 1•2 tsp honey (optional)

Instructions:

1. In a small bowl, combine the cottage cheese and diced pineapple.

2. If desired, drizzle 1•2 tsp of honey over the top.

3. Gently stir the mixture to combine.

4. Serve chilled or at room temperature.

Tips:
- Use low•fat or non•fat cottage cheese to keep the calorie and fat content lower.

- Choose fresh or canned pineapple packed in its own juice, not heavy syrup.

- Start with a small portion, like 1/2 cup cottage cheese and 1/4 cup pineapple.

- The honey is optional, as the pineapple provides natural sweetness.

- Portion the cottage cheese and pineapple into individual servings for easy meal prep.

This cottage cheese and pineapple snack provides a good source of protein, fiber, and vitamins. The soft, smooth texture of the cottage cheese and the juicy pineapple make it an easy•to•digest option after gastric bypass surgery. Adjust the portion sizes as needed to meet your individual dietary needs.

57. Smoothie Bowls (with protein powder)

Ingredients:

- 1/4 cup chia seeds
- 1 cup unsweetened almond milk or low•fat milk
- 1/4 tsp vanilla extract (optional)
- Pinch of cinnamon (optional)

Instructions:

1. In a medium bowl or mason jar, combine the chia seeds, milk, vanilla (if using), and cinnamon (if using). Stir well to combine.

2. Cover the bowl or seal the jar and refrigerate for at least 2 hours, or up to 5 days, stirring occasionally. The chia seeds will thicken the mixture into a pudding•like consistency.

3. When ready to serve, give the pudding a final stir to incorporate any remaining chia seeds.

4. Portion the chia seed pudding into individual servings.

Tips:
- Use unsweetened almond milk or low•fat dairy milk for a creamier texture.

- The vanilla and cinnamon are optional, but can add a bit of flavor.

- Avoid adding any sweeteners, as the goal is an unsweetened pudding.

- Portion the pudding into individual servings for easy meal prep.

- Top with fresh or frozen berries, if desired.

This unsweetened chia seed pudding provides a nutrient•dense, high•fiber snack or breakfast option that is easy to digest after gastric bypass surgery. The smooth, pudding•like texture makes it a great choice for post•op meal prep.

58. Chia Seed Pudding (unsweetened)

Ingredients:

• 1/4 cup chia seeds
• 1 cup unsweetened almond milk or low•fat milk
• 1/4 tsp vanilla extract (optional)
• Pinch of cinnamon (optional)

Instructions:

1. In a medium bowl or mason jar, combine the chia seeds, milk, vanilla (if using), and cinnamon (if using). Stir well to combine.

2. Cover the bowl or seal the jar and refrigerate for at least 2 hours, or up to 5 days, stirring occasionally. The chia seeds will thicken the mixture into a pudding•like consistency.

3. When ready to serve, give the pudding a final stir to incorporate any remaining chia seeds.

4. Portion the chia seed pudding into individual servings.

Tips:
• Use unsweetened almond milk or low•fat dairy milk for a creamier texture.

• The vanilla and cinnamon are optional, but can add a bit of flavor.

• Avoid adding any sweeteners, as the goal is an unsweetened pudding.

• Portion the pudding into individual servings for easy meal prep.

• Top with fresh or frozen berries, if desired.

This unsweetened chia seed pudding provides a nutrient•dense, high•fiber snack or breakfast option that is easy to digest after gastric bypass surgery. The smooth, pudding•like texture makes it a great choice for post•op meal prep.

59. Overnight Oats (with almond milk)

Ingredients:

- 1/2 cup old•fashioned rolled oats
- 1 cup unsweetened almond milk
- 1 tbsp chia seeds (optional)
- 1/2 tsp vanilla extract (optional)
- Pinch of cinnamon (optional)

Instructions:

1. In a medium bowl or mason jar, combine the rolled oats, almond milk, chia seeds (if using), vanilla (if using), and cinnamon (if using). Stir well to mix.

2. Cover the bowl or seal the jar and refrigerate overnight, or for at least 4 hours.

3. When ready to serve, give the overnight oats a stir to incorporate any remaining liquid.

4. Portion the overnight oats into individual servings.

Tips:
- Use old•fashioned rolled oats, not instant oats, for a creamier texture.

- Unsweetened almond milk provides a creamy base without added sugars.

- The chia seeds, vanilla, and cinnamon are optional additions for extra flavor.

- Avoid adding any sweeteners, as the goal is an unsweetened breakfast.

- Top with fresh or frozen berries, if desired.

- Portion the overnight oats into individual servings for easy meal prep.

This overnight oats recipe made with almond milk provides a nutrient•dense, high•fiber breakfast that is easy to digest after gastric bypass surgery. The soft, creamy texture makes it a great option for post•op meal prep.

60. Quinoa Porridge

Ingredients:

- 1/2 cup uncooked quinoa, rinsed
- 1 cup low•fat milk or unsweetened almond milk
- 1/4 tsp vanilla extract (optional)
- 1/4 tsp ground cinnamon (optional)
- Pinch of salt

Instructions:

1. In a small saucepan, combine the rinsed quinoa and milk. Bring the mixture to a boil over medium•high heat.

2. Once boiling, reduce the heat to low, cover the pan, and simmer for 15•20 minutes, stirring occasionally, until the quinoa is very soft and the porridge has thickened.

3. Remove the pan from heat and stir in the vanilla (if using), cinnamon (if using), and a pinch of salt.

4. Serve the quinoa porridge warm, portioning it into individual servings.

Tips:
- Use low•fat dairy milk or unsweetened almond milk for a creamy texture.

- The vanilla and cinnamon are optional additions for extra flavor.

- Avoid adding any sweeteners, as the goal is an unsweetened porridge.

- Top with fresh or frozen berries, if desired.

- Portion the quinoa porridge into individual servings for easy meal prep.

This quinoa porridge provides a nutrient•dense, high•protein breakfast option that is easy to digest after gastric bypass surgery. The soft, creamy texture makes it a great choice for post•op meal prep. Adjust the cooking time as needed to achieve the desired consistency.

61. Chicken Salad (with Greek yogurt)

Ingredients:

- 2 cups cooked, shredded or diced chicken breast
- 1/2 cup plain, unsweetened Greek yogurt
- 2 tbsp finely diced celery
- 2 tbsp finely diced onion
- 1 tsp Dijon mustard
- 1/4 tsp dried dill (optional)
- Salt and pepper to taste

Instructions:

1. In a medium bowl, combine the cooked, shredded or diced chicken, Greek yogurt, celery, onion, Dijon mustard, and dried dill (if using).

2. Stir the ingredients together until well mixed.

3. Season the chicken salad with a small amount of salt and pepper to taste.

4. Serve the chicken salad chilled or at room temperature.

Tips:
- Use plain, unsweetened Greek yogurt for a higher protein content.

- Adjust the amount of yogurt to your desired consistency.

- Finely dice the celery and onion for a smooth texture.

- The dried dill is optional, but adds a nice flavor.

- Portion the chicken salad into individual servings for easy meal prep.

This chicken salad made with Greek yogurt provides a protein•rich, easy•to•digest option for meal prep after gastric bypass surgery. The smooth, creamy texture makes it a great choice for post•op meals. Serve it on its own or use it as a topping for soft, cooked vegetables.

62. Turkey Wrap (lettuce wrap)

Ingredients:

• 4•6 large lettuce leaves (such as romaine or butter lettuce)
• 4 oz sliced turkey breast
• 2 tbsp hummus or Greek yogurt•based dressing
• 1/4 cup diced cucumber
• 1/4 cup diced tomato
• 1 tbsp finely chopped red onion (optional)
• Salt and pepper to taste

Instructions:

1. Rinse the lettuce leaves and pat them dry.

2. Lay the lettuce leaves flat on a clean surface.

3. Spread 1•2 tbsp of hummus or dressing down the center of each lettuce leaf.

4. Top the hummus/dressing with slices of turkey breast.

5. Add the diced cucumber, tomato, and red onion (if using) on top of the turkey.

6. Season with a small amount of salt and pepper.

7. Carefully wrap the lettuce around the fillings, tucking in the sides as you go.

8. Serve the turkey lettuce wraps immediately or refrigerate for meal prep.

Tips:
• Choose large, sturdy lettuce leaves for easy wrapping.

• Adjust the fillings to your taste preferences.

• Portion the wrapped lettuce leaves into individual servings for easy meal prep.

• Refrigerate wrapped lettuce leaves for up to 3•4 days.

This turkey lettuce wrap provides a low•carb, easy•to•digest option for a post•gastric bypass meal or snack. The soft lettuce leaves and simple fillings make it a great choice for meal prep.

63. Egg Salad (with light mayo)

Ingredients:

- 6 hard•boiled eggs, peeled and chopped
- 2 tbsp light mayonnaise
- 1 tbsp finely diced celery
- 1 tbsp finely diced onion
- 1 tsp Dijon mustard
- 1/4 tsp dried dill (optional)
- Salt and pepper to taste

Instructions:

1. In a medium bowl, combine the chopped hard•boiled eggs, light mayonnaise, diced celery, diced onion, Dijon mustard, and dried dill (if using).

2. Stir the ingredients together until well mixed.

3. Season the egg salad with a small amount of salt and pepper to taste.

4. Serve the egg salad chilled or at room temperature.

Tips:
- Use light or low•fat mayonnaise to reduce the calorie and fat content.

- Finely dice the celery and onion for a smooth texture.

- The dried dill is optional, but adds a nice flavor.

- Adjust the amount of mayonnaise to your desired consistency.

- Portion the egg salad into individual servings for easy meal prep.

This egg salad made with light mayonnaise provides a protein•rich, easy•to•digest option for meal prep after gastric bypass surgery. The smooth, creamy texture makes it a great choice for post•op meals. Serve it on its own or use it as a topping for soft, cooked vegetables.

64. Vegetable Soup (chunky)

Ingredients:

- 2 tbsp olive oil
- 1 onion, diced
- 2 carrots, peeled and diced
- 2 celery stalks, diced
- 2 cloves garlic, minced
- 4 cups low•sodium vegetable or chicken broth
- 1 (15 oz) can diced tomatoes
- 1 cup frozen peas
- 1 cup frozen green beans
- 1 tsp dried thyme
- 1/2 tsp dried oregano
- Salt and pepper to taste

Instructions:

1. In a large pot or Dutch oven, heat the olive oil over medium heat.

2. Add the diced onion, carrots, and celery. Sauté for 5•7 minutes, until the vegetables are softened.

3. Add the minced garlic and sauté for 1 minute until fragrant.

4. Pour in the vegetable or chicken broth and the can of diced tomatoes. Stir to combine.

5. Add the frozen peas, green beans, dried thyme, and dried oregano. Season with a small amount of salt and pepper.

6. Bring the soup to a boil, then reduce heat and let simmer for 15•20 minutes, until the vegetables are tender. Serve the chunky vegetable soup warm, portioning it into individual servings.

Tips:
- Use low•sodium broth to control salt intake.
- Adjust the vegetable amounts and types to your preferences.
- The soup can be blended partially or fully for a smoother texture, if desired.
- Portion the soup into individual servings for easy meal prep.

This chunky vegetable soup provides a nutrient•dense, easy•to•digest option for meal prep after gastric bypass surgery. The soft, cooked vegetables and flavorful broth make it a comforting and satisfying choice.

65. Stuffed Bell Peppers (quinoa, lean meat)

Ingredients:

- 4 bell peppers, halved and seeded
- 1/2 lb lean ground turkey or ground chicken
- 1/2 cup cooked quinoa
- 1/4 cup diced onion
- 1 clove garlic, minced
- 1 tsp dried oregano
- 1/4 tsp red pepper flakes (optional)
- Salt and pepper to taste
- 1/4 cup shredded low•fat mozzarella cheese (optional)

Instructions:

1. Preheat oven to 375°F. Lightly grease a baking dish.

2. In a skillet over medium heat, cook the ground turkey/chicken until no longer pink, 5•7 minutes. Drain any excess fat.

3. In a bowl, combine the cooked ground meat, cooked quinoa, diced onion, minced garlic, dried oregano, and red pepper flakes (if using). Season with a small amount of salt and pepper.

4. Stuff the mixture into the hollowed•out bell pepper halves and place them in the prepared baking dish.

5. If using, sprinkle the shredded mozzarella cheese over the top of the stuffed peppers.

6. Bake for 20•25 minutes, until the peppers are tender and the filling is heated through.

7. Let the stuffed peppers cool slightly before serving or portioning out.

Tips:
- Use lean ground turkey or chicken to keep the fat content low.
- Adjust the amount of quinoa and meat to your preference.
- The mozzarella cheese is optional, but adds a nice creamy element.
- Portion the stuffed peppers into individual servings for easy meal prep.

These stuffed bell peppers provide a nutrient•dense, protein•rich meal that is easy to digest after gastric bypass surgery. The soft, cooked peppers and quinoa•meat filling make it a great option for post•op meal prep.

66. Tuna Salad (with light mayo)

Ingredients:

- 2 (5 oz) cans of tuna, drained
- 2 tbsp light mayonnaise
- 1 tbsp finely diced celery
- 1 tbsp finely diced onion
- 1 tsp Dijon mustard
- 1/4 tsp dried dill (optional)
- Salt and pepper to taste

Instructions:

1. In a medium bowl, combine the drained tuna, light mayonnaise, diced celery, diced onion, Dijon mustard, and dried dill (if using).

2. Stir the ingredients together until well mixed.

3. Season the tuna salad with a small amount of salt and pepper to taste.

4. Serve the tuna salad chilled or at room temperature.

Tips:
- Use light or low•fat mayonnaise to reduce the calorie and fat content.

- Finely dice the celery and onion for a smooth texture.

- The dried dill is optional, but adds a nice flavor.

- Adjust the amount of mayonnaise to your desired consistency.

- Portion the tuna salad into individual servings for easy meal prep.

This tuna salad made with light mayonnaise provides a protein•rich, easy•to•digest option for meal prep after gastric bypass surgery. The smooth, creamy texture makes it a great choice for post•op meals. Serve it on its own or use it as a topping for soft, cooked vegetables.

67. Salmon Salad (with avocado)

Ingredients:

- 1 (5 oz) can of salmon, drained and flaked
- 1/2 avocado, diced
- 2 tbsp plain Greek yogurt
- 1 tbsp lemon juice
- 1 tsp Dijon mustard
- 1 tbsp finely diced celery
- 1 tbsp finely diced onion
- Salt and pepper to taste

Instructions:

1. In a medium bowl, combine the flaked salmon, diced avocado, Greek yogurt, lemon juice, Dijon mustard, diced celery, and diced onion.

2. Gently mix the ingredients together until well combined.

3. Season the salmon salad with a small amount of salt and pepper to taste.

4. Serve the salmon salad chilled or at room temperature.

Tips:
- Use canned salmon for convenience, or bake/grill fresh salmon and flake it.

- The Greek yogurt provides a creamy texture without the high fat content of mayonnaise.

- Finely dice the celery and onion for a smooth texture.

- Adjust the amount of Greek yogurt to your desired consistency.

- Portion the salmon salad into individual servings for easy meal prep.

This salmon salad with avocado provides a nutrient•dense, easy•to•digest option for meal prep after gastric bypass surgery. The healthy fats from the salmon and avocado, combined with the protein•rich Greek yogurt, make it a satisfying choice.

68. Shrimp Cocktail (low•sodium sauce)

Ingredients:

- 1 lb cooked, peeled and deveined shrimp
- 1/4 cup low•sodium ketchup
- 1 tbsp lemon juice
- 1 tsp prepared horseradish
- 1/4 tsp Worcestershire sauce
- 1/4 tsp garlic powder
- 1/8 tsp cayenne pepper (optional)
- Salt and pepper to taste

Instructions:

1. In a small bowl, combine the low•sodium ketchup, lemon juice, horseradish, Worcestershire sauce, garlic powder, and cayenne pepper (if using). Stir to mix well.

2. Arrange the cooked shrimp on a serving platter or in individual dishes.

3. Serve the shrimp cocktail chilled, with the low•sodium sauce on the side for dipping.

Tips:
- Use cooked, peeled and deveined shrimp for easy prep.

- Choose a low•sodium ketchup to reduce the overall sodium content.

- Adjust the amount of horseradish and cayenne to your taste preferences.

- Portion the shrimp and sauce into individual servings for easy meal prep.

- Refrigerate the shrimp and sauce separately until ready to serve.

This shrimp cocktail with a low•sodium sauce provides a protein•rich, easy•to•digest option that is well•suited for meal prep after gastric bypass surgery. The cool, refreshing flavors make it a great choice for a light snack or appetizer.

69. Veggie Burger (without bun)

Ingredients:

- 1 (15 oz) can black beans, rinsed and drained
- 1/2 cup cooked quinoa
- 1/4 cup rolled oats
- 1 egg, lightly beaten
- 2 tbsp finely diced onion
- 1 clove garlic, minced
- 1 tsp chili powder
- 1/2 tsp cumin
- 1/4 tsp salt
- 1/4 tsp black pepper

Instructions:

1. In a medium bowl, mash the rinsed and drained black beans with a fork or potato masher.

2. Add the cooked quinoa, rolled oats, egg, diced onion, minced garlic, chili powder, cumin, salt, and pepper. Mix well until fully combined.

3. Form the mixture into 4•6 patties, about 1/2 inch thick.

4. Heat a nonstick skillet over medium heat. Cook the veggie patties for 3•4 minutes per side, until lightly browned.

5. Serve the veggie burgers warm, without a bun. Top with desired toppings like avocado, tomato, or a dollop of Greek yogurt.

Tips:
- The quinoa and oats help bind the veggie patties together.

- Finely dice the onion for a smoother texture.

- Adjust seasoning to your taste preferences.

- Portion the cooked veggie burgers into individual servings for easy meal prep. Reheat gently before serving.

This veggie burger without a bun provides a nutrient•dense, high•fiber option that is easy to digest after gastric bypass surgery. The soft, patty•like texture makes it a great choice for post•op meals.

70. Lentil Salad

Ingredients:

- 1 cup dry brown or green lentils, rinsed
- 3 cups vegetable or chicken broth
- 1 red bell pepper, diced
- 1 cucumber, diced
- 1/2 red onion, finely chopped
- 1/4 cup chopped fresh parsley
- 2 tbsp chopped fresh mint (optional)
- 2 tbsp olive oil
- 2 tbsp red wine vinegar
- 1 tsp Dijon mustard
- 1 garlic clove, minced
- 1/2 tsp salt
- 1/4 tsp black pepper

Instructions:

1. In a medium saucepan, combine the lentils and broth. Bring to a boil over high heat. Reduce heat to low, cover and simmer for 15•20 minutes, until lentils are tender. Drain any excess liquid and let cool.

2. In a large bowl, combine the cooked lentils, bell pepper, cucumber, red onion, parsley, and mint (if using).

3. In a small bowl, whisk together the olive oil, vinegar, mustard, garlic, salt, and pepper.

4. Pour the dressing over the lentil salad and toss gently to coat.

5. Refrigerate the lentil salad for at least 30 minutes to allow the flavors to meld.

6. Serve chilled or at room temperature. This salad can be made a day in advance.

The lentils provide protein and fiber, while the fresh vegetables and herbs add crunch and flavor. This lentil salad makes a great side dish or light main course. It's perfect for picnics, potlucks, or a healthy lunch.

71. Grilled Chicken Breast (herbs)

Ingredients:

- 4 boneless, skinless chicken breasts
- 2 tbsp olive oil
- 2 tbsp chopped fresh herbs (such as rosemary, thyme, oregano, or parsley)
- 1 tsp garlic powder
- 1 tsp onion powder
- 1/2 tsp salt
- 1/4 tsp black pepper

Instructions:

1. Preheat your grill or grill pan to medium•high heat.

2. In a shallow dish or resealable plastic bag, combine the olive oil, chopped fresh herbs, garlic powder, onion powder, salt, and pepper. Add the chicken breasts and turn to coat them evenly in the herb mixture.

3. Grill the chicken for 5•7 minutes per side, or until the internal temperature reaches 165°F. The chicken should be cooked through and no longer pink in the center.

4. Transfer the grilled chicken breasts to a clean plate or cutting board. Let them rest for 5 minutes before serving.

5. Serve the grilled herb chicken breasts warm. They pair well with roasted vegetables, a fresh salad, or your choice of side dishes.

The combination of fresh herbs, garlic, and onion creates a flavorful marinade that infuses the chicken with delicious flavor as it grills. This is a simple and healthy grilled chicken recipe that's perfect for a weeknight dinner or summer barbecue.

72. Baked Salmon (lemon, dill)

Ingredients:

- 4 salmon fillets (about 1 lb total)
- 2 tbsp olive oil
- 2 tbsp freshly squeezed lemon juice
- 1 tsp grated lemon zest
- 2 tsp dried dill
- 1/2 tsp garlic powder
- 1/4 tsp salt
- 1/4 tsp black pepper

Instructions:

1. Preheat the oven to 400°F. Lightly grease a baking dish or line with parchment paper.

2. In a small bowl, whisk together the olive oil, lemon juice, lemon zest, dill, garlic powder, salt, and pepper.

3. Place the salmon fillets in the prepared baking dish. Pour the lemon•dill mixture over the top, making sure to coat the fish evenly.

4. Bake for 12•15 minutes, or until the salmon is opaque and flakes easily with a fork and reaches an internal temperature of 145°F.

5. Serve the baked salmon immediately, garnished with extra lemon wedges and fresh dill if desired. Enjoy!

The bright lemon and fragrant dill flavors pair beautifully with the rich salmon. This is a simple yet elegant baked salmon recipe that's perfect for a healthy and delicious meal.

73. Turkey Meatloaf

Ingredients:

- 1 lb ground turkey
- 1 cup breadcrumbs
- 1/2 cup milk
- 1 egg
- 1/2 onion, finely chopped
- 2 cloves garlic, minced
- 1 tsp dried thyme
- 1 tsp dried oregano
- 1/2 tsp salt
- 1/4 tsp black pepper
- 1/4 cup ketchup or tomato sauce

Instructions:

1. Preheat the oven to 375°F. Lightly grease a 9x5 inch loaf pan.

2. In a large bowl, combine the ground turkey, breadcrumbs, milk, egg, onion, garlic, thyme, oregano, salt, and pepper. Mix well until all the ingredients are evenly distributed.

3. Transfer the turkey mixture to the prepared loaf pan and shape it into a loaf.

4. Spread the ketchup or tomato sauce evenly over the top of the meatloaf.

5. Bake for 55•60 minutes, or until the internal temperature reaches 165°F.

6. Let the meatloaf rest for 5•10 minutes before slicing and serving.

Serve the turkey meatloaf warm, with your choice of sides like mashed potatoes, roasted vegetables, or a fresh salad. The ketchup or tomato sauce on top adds a nice tangy glaze to the meatloaf.

This turkey meatloaf is a healthier alternative to traditional beef meatloaf, but still full of flavor. It's a comforting and easy•to•make main dish.

74. Stir•fried Tofu (with veggies)

Ingredients:

- 1 block (14 oz) extra•firm tofu, cubed
- 2 tbsp vegetable or peanut oil
- 1 cup sliced mushrooms
- 1 cup broccoli florets
- 1 red bell pepper, sliced
- 1 cup snow peas or snap peas
- 3 cloves garlic, minced
- 1 tbsp grated fresh ginger
- 2 tbsp low•sodium soy sauce
- 1 tbsp rice vinegar
- 1 tsp sesame oil
- 1/4 tsp red pepper flakes (optional)
- Salt and pepper to taste
- Cooked rice, for serving

Instructions:

1. Press the tofu for 15•30 minutes to remove excess moisture. Cut into 1•inch cubes.

2. Heat the vegetable oil in a large skillet or wok over medium•high heat. Add the tofu cubes and cook, turning occasionally, until golden brown on all sides, about 5•7 minutes. Transfer to a plate.

3. Add the mushrooms, broccoli, bell pepper, and snow peas to the skillet. Stir•fry for 3•4 minutes until the vegetables are crisp•tender.

4. Add the garlic and ginger and cook for 1 minute, until fragrant.

5. Return the tofu to the skillet. Add the soy sauce, rice vinegar, sesame oil, and red pepper flakes (if using). Toss everything together and cook for 2•3 minutes more.

6. Season with salt and pepper to taste.

7. Serve the stir•fried tofu and vegetables immediately over steamed rice.

This stir•fry is packed with fresh vegetables and protein•rich tofu. The soy sauce, ginger, and sesame oil create a delicious savory sauce that coats everything. It's a quick and healthy vegetarian main dish.

75. Stuffed Zucchini Boats (lean meat)

Ingredients:

- 4 medium zucchini, halved lengthwise
- 1 lb lean ground turkey or ground chicken
- 1/2 onion, finely chopped
- 2 cloves garlic, minced
- 1 cup diced tomatoes
- 1/2 cup cooked brown rice
- 1/4 cup grated Parmesan cheese
- 2 tbsp chopped fresh basil
- 1 tsp dried oregano
- 1/4 tsp red pepper flakes (optional)
- Salt and pepper to taste
- 1/2 cup shredded mozzarella cheese

Instructions:

1. Preheat the oven to 375°F. Scoop out the flesh from the zucchini halves, leaving about 1/4 inch of the shell. Finely chop the zucchini flesh.

2. In a skillet over medium heat, cook the ground turkey or chicken, onion, and garlic until the meat is browned and cooked through, 5•7 minutes. Drain any excess fat.

3. Add the chopped zucchini flesh, diced tomatoes, cooked rice, Parmesan, basil, oregano, and red pepper flakes (if using). Season with salt and pepper.

4. Stuff the zucchini boats evenly with the meat and vegetable mixture.

5. Place the stuffed zucchini boats in a baking dish. Top with the shredded mozzarella cheese.

6. Bake for 20•25 minutes, until the zucchini is tender and the cheese is melted and bubbly.

7. Serve the stuffed zucchini boats warm. Enjoy!

These stuffed zucchini boats are a healthy and delicious way to enjoy lean ground meat and fresh vegetables. The Parmesan and mozzarella cheeses add a nice creamy texture.

76. Spaghetti Squash (with marinara)

Ingredients:

• 1 medium spaghetti squash, halved lengthwise and seeded
• 1 cup low•sodium marinara sauce
• 2 tbsp grated Parmesan cheese (optional)
• Fresh basil leaves, chopped (optional)
• Salt and pepper to taste

Instructions:

1. Preheat the oven to 400°F. Line a baking sheet with parchment paper.

2. Place the spaghetti squash halves cut•side down on the prepared baking sheet. Roast for 30•40 minutes, until the squash is very tender when pierced with a fork.

3. Remove the spaghetti squash from the oven and let cool slightly. Use a fork to gently scrape the flesh into long, spaghetti•like strands.

4. In a medium saucepan, heat the low•sodium marinara sauce over medium heat until warmed through.

5. Divide the spaghetti squash strands into individual servings and top with the warm marinara sauce.

6. If desired, sprinkle a small amount of grated Parmesan cheese and chopped fresh basil over the top.

7. Serve the spaghetti squash with marinara warm.

Tips:
• Choose a low•sodium marinara sauce to control sodium intake.
• The Parmesan cheese and fresh basil are optional toppings.
• Portion the spaghetti squash and marinara into individual servings for easy meal prep.
• Reheat gently before serving.

This spaghetti squash with marinara sauce provides a low•carb, nutrient•dense option that is easy to digest after gastric bypass surgery. The soft, noodle•like texture of the spaghetti squash makes it a great substitute for traditional pasta.

77. Grilled Shrimp (garlic, lemon)

Ingredients:

- 1 lb large shrimp, peeled and deveined
- 3 tbsp olive oil
- 3 cloves garlic, minced
- 2 tbsp freshly squeezed lemon juice
- 1 tsp grated lemon zest
- 1/4 tsp red pepper flakes (optional)
- 1/2 tsp salt
- 1/4 tsp black pepper

Instructions:

1. In a large bowl, combine the shrimp, olive oil, minced garlic, lemon juice, lemon zest, red pepper flakes (if using), salt, and black pepper. Toss to coat the shrimp evenly.

2. Preheat your grill or grill pan to medium•high heat.

3. Thread the marinated shrimp onto metal or wooden skewers, leaving a little space between each shrimp.

4. Grill the shrimp skewers for 2•3 minutes per side, until the shrimp are opaque and cooked through.

5. Serve the grilled garlic lemon shrimp immediately, garnished with extra lemon wedges if desired.

The combination of garlic, lemon, and a touch of heat from the red pepper flakes creates a delicious flavor profile for the grilled shrimp. This recipe is quick and easy, making it perfect for a summer barbecue or weeknight dinner.

Serve the shrimp with grilled vegetables, over a salad, or alongside rice or pasta for a complete meal. Enjoy!

78. Turkey Chili

Ingredients:

- 1 lb ground turkey
- 1 onion, diced
- 3 cloves garlic, minced
- 2 tbsp chili powder
- 1 tbsp ground cumin
- 1 tsp dried oregano
- 1/2 tsp smoked paprika
- 1/4 tsp cayenne pepper (optional, for heat)
- 1 can (15 oz) diced tomatoes
- 1 can (15 oz) kidney beans, drained and rinsed
- 1 can (15 oz) black beans, drained and rinsed
- 1 cup low•sodium chicken or vegetable broth
- Salt and black pepper to taste
- Toppings: shredded cheese, diced avocado, chopped onion, sour cream, etc.

Instructions:

1. In a large pot or Dutch oven, cook the ground turkey over medium•high heat, breaking it up with a wooden spoon, until browned and cooked through, about 5•7 minutes. Drain any excess fat.

2. Add the diced onion and minced garlic to the pot. Cook for 2•3 minutes until the onion is translucent.

3. Stir in the chili powder, cumin, oregano, smoked paprika, and cayenne (if using). Cook for 1 minute to toast the spices.

4. Pour in the diced tomatoes, kidney beans, black beans, and chicken/vegetable broth. Stir to combine.

5. Bring the chili to a simmer and let it cook for 20•25 minutes, stirring occasionally, until thickened.

6. Season with salt and black pepper to taste.

7. Serve the turkey chili hot, topped with your desired toppings.

This turkey chili is a healthier alternative to traditional beef chili, but still full of bold, spicy flavor. It's a comforting and satisfying meal, especially on a cool day.

79. Quinoa and Vegetable Stir•fry

Ingredients:

- 1 cup cooked quinoa
- 1 tbsp olive oil
- 1 cup chopped broccoli florets
- 1 cup sliced mushrooms
- 1/2 cup diced bell pepper
- 1/2 cup diced zucchini
- 2 cloves garlic, minced
- 1 tsp grated fresh ginger
- 2 tbsp low•sodium soy sauce or tamari
- 1 tsp sesame oil (optional)
- Salt and pepper to taste

Instructions:

1. In a large skillet or wok, heat the olive oil over medium•high heat.

2. Add the chopped broccoli, sliced mushrooms, diced bell pepper, and diced zucchini. Stir•fry for 5•7 minutes, until the vegetables are tender•crisp.

3. Add the minced garlic and grated ginger. Stir•fry for 1 minute until fragrant.

4. Stir in the cooked quinoa, low•sodium soy sauce or tamari, and sesame oil (if using). Toss everything together until well combined.

5. Season the quinoa and vegetable stir•fry with a small amount of salt and pepper to taste.

6. Serve the stir•fry warm, portioning it into individual servings.

Tips:
- Use a variety of colorful, nutrient•dense vegetables.
- Adjust the vegetable amounts to your preference.
- The sesame oil adds a nice flavor, but is optional.
- Portion the stir•fry into individual servings for easy meal prep.
- Reheat gently before serving.

This quinoa and vegetable stir•fry provides a nutrient•dense, high•fiber meal that is easy to digest after gastric bypass surgery. The soft, tender vegetables and quinoa make it a great option for post•op meal prep.

80. Baked Cod (with herbs)

Ingredients:

- 4 cod fillets (about 1 lb total)
- 2 tbsp olive oil
- 2 tbsp chopped fresh parsley
- 1 tbsp chopped fresh dill
- 1 tbsp chopped fresh thyme
- 2 cloves garlic, minced
- 1/2 tsp paprika
- 1/4 tsp salt
- 1/4 tsp black pepper
- Lemon wedges for serving

Instructions:

1. Preheat the oven to 400°F. Lightly grease a baking dish or line it with parchment paper.

2. In a small bowl, mix together the olive oil, parsley, dill, thyme, garlic, paprika, salt, and pepper.

3. Place the cod fillets in the prepared baking dish. Spoon the herb mixture evenly over the top of the fish, making sure to coat it completely.

4. Bake for 12•15 minutes, or until the cod is opaque and flakes easily with a fork. The internal temperature should reach 145°F.

5. Serve the baked cod immediately, garnished with lemon wedges.

The combination of fresh herbs, garlic, and paprika creates a flavorful crust on the tender, flaky cod. This is a simple yet delicious way to prepare cod that highlights the natural flavors of the fish.

Serve the baked cod with roasted vegetables, a fresh salad, or your choice of sides for a complete and healthy meal. Enjoy!

81. Chicken Stir•fry (with broccoli)

Ingredients:

- 1 lb boneless, skinless chicken breasts, cut into 1•inch pieces
- 2 tbsp vegetable or peanut oil
- 3 cups broccoli florets
- 1 red bell pepper, sliced
- 3 cloves garlic, minced
- 1 tbsp grated fresh ginger
- 2 tbsp low•sodium soy sauce
- 1 tbsp rice vinegar
- 1 tsp sesame oil
- 1/4 tsp red pepper flakes (optional)
- Salt and pepper to taste
- Cooked rice, for serving

Instructions:

1. Heat the vegetable oil in a large skillet or wok over high heat.

2. Add the chicken and stir•fry for 3•4 minutes, until the chicken is lightly browned but not fully cooked through.

3. Add the broccoli florets and bell pepper slices to the skillet. Stir•fry for 3•4 minutes, until the vegetables are crisp•tender.

4. Push the chicken and vegetables to the sides of the skillet. Add the minced garlic and grated ginger to the center of the skillet. Cook for 1 minute, until fragrant.

5. Stir the garlic and ginger into the chicken and vegetables.

6. Add the soy sauce, rice vinegar, sesame oil, and red pepper flakes (if using). Toss everything together and cook for 2•3 minutes more, until the chicken is cooked through.

7. Season with salt and pepper to taste.

8. Serve the chicken stir•fry immediately over steamed rice.

This chicken and broccoli stir•fry is a quick and healthy weeknight meal. The combination of tender chicken, crisp broccoli, and a savory sauce makes for a delicious and balanced dish.

82. Vegetable Lasagna (zucchini noodles)

Ingredients:

- 1 (6 oz) can tomato paste
- 1 tsp dried oregano
- 1/2 tsp dried basil
- 1/4 tsp red pepper flakes (optional)
- Salt and pepper to taste
- 1 (15 oz) container part•skim ricotta cheese
- 1 cup shredded mozzarella cheese
- 1/4 cup grated Parmesan cheese

- 3 medium zucchinis, sliced lengthwise into thin noodle•like strips
- 1 tbsp olive oil
- 1 onion, diced
- 3 cloves garlic, minced
- 8 oz sliced mushrooms
- 1 red bell pepper, diced
- 1 cup baby spinach leaves
- 1 (15 oz) can diced tomatoes

Instructions:

1. Preheat the oven to 375°F. Lightly grease a 9x13 inch baking dish.

2. In a large skillet, heat the olive oil over medium heat. Add the onion and garlic and cook for 2•3 minutes until fragrant.

3. Add the mushrooms and bell pepper to the skillet. Cook for 5•7 minutes, until the vegetables are tender.

4. Stir in the baby spinach, diced tomatoes, tomato paste, oregano, basil, and red pepper flakes (if using). Season with salt and pepper.

5. In a separate bowl, mix together the ricotta, 1/2 cup of the mozzarella, and the Parmesan cheese.

6. Arrange a layer of zucchini noodles in the bottom of the prepared baking dish. Top with half of the vegetable mixture, then half of the ricotta cheese mixture.

7. Repeat the layers of zucchini noodles, vegetables, and ricotta cheese.

8. Top the lasagna with the remaining 1/2 cup of mozzarella cheese.

9. Bake for 30•35 minutes, until the cheese is melted and bubbly.

10. Let the lasagna cool for 5•10 minutes before slicing and serving.

This vegetable lasagna uses zucchini noodles instead of traditional pasta for a lighter, low•carb option. It's packed with fresh veggies and creamy ricotta cheese.

83. Lean Beef Stir•fry (with bell peppers)

Ingredients:

- 1 lb lean beef (such as sirloin or flank steak), thinly sliced
- 1 tbsp olive oil
- 1 red bell pepper, sliced
- 1 yellow bell pepper, sliced
- 1 clove garlic, minced
- 1 tsp grated fresh ginger
- 2 tbsp low•sodium soy sauce or tamari
- 1 tsp sesame oil (optional)
- Salt and pepper to taste

Instructions:

1. In a large skillet or wok, heat the olive oil over high heat.

2. Add the thinly sliced beef and stir•fry for 2•3 minutes, until the beef is lightly browned but still slightly pink.

3. Add the sliced red and yellow bell peppers, minced garlic, and grated ginger. Stir•fry for an additional 3•4 minutes, until the vegetables are tender•crisp.

4. Stir in the low•sodium soy sauce or tamari, and the sesame oil (if using). Toss everything together until well combined.

5. Season the beef and vegetable stir•fry with a small amount of salt and pepper to taste.

6. Serve the stir•fry warm, portioning it into individual servings.

Tips:
- Use lean cuts of beef, such as sirloin or flank steak, to minimize fat content.
- Slice the beef thinly across the grain for a more tender texture.
- Adjust the vegetable amounts to your preference.
- The sesame oil adds a nice flavor, but is optional.
- Portion the stir•fry into individual servings for easy meal prep.
- Reheat gently before serving.

This lean beef and bell pepper stir•fry provides a protein•rich, easy•to•digest meal option for meal prep after gastric bypass surgery. The tender beef and crisp•tender vegetables make it a satisfying and nutritious choice.

84. Chicken Cacciatore

Ingredients:

- 1 lb boneless, skinless chicken breasts, cut into 1•inch pieces
- 1 tbsp olive oil
- 1 onion, diced
- 2 cloves garlic, minced
- 1 (14.5 oz) can diced tomatoes
- 1/2 cup low•sodium chicken broth
- 1 tsp dried oregano
- 1/2 tsp dried basil
- 1/4 tsp red pepper flakes (optional)
- Salt and pepper to taste

Instructions:

1. In a large skillet or Dutch oven, heat the olive oil over medium•high heat.

2. Add the diced chicken pieces and cook for 3•4 minutes, until lightly browned on all sides.

3. Add the diced onion and minced garlic to the pan. Sauté for 2•3 minutes until the onion is translucent.

4. Pour in the can of diced tomatoes and the low•sodium chicken broth. Stir in the dried oregano, dried basil, and red pepper flakes (if using).

5. Bring the mixture to a simmer, then reduce heat to medium•low. Let the cacciatore simmer for 15•20 minutes, until the chicken is cooked through and the sauce has thickened slightly.

6. Season the chicken cacciatore with a small amount of salt and pepper to taste.

7. Serve the cacciatore warm, portioning it into individual servings.

Tips:
- Use boneless, skinless chicken breasts to keep the dish lean.
- Adjust the amount of red pepper flakes to your spice preference.
- Serve the cacciatore over mashed cauliflower or zucchini noodles for a low•carb option.
- Portion the cacciatore into individual servings for easy meal prep.
- Reheat gently before serving.

This chicken cacciatore provides a flavorful, protein•rich meal that is easy to digest after gastric bypass surgery. The tender chicken and vegetable•based sauce make it a great choice for post•op meal prep.

85. Baked Tilapia (with lemon)

Ingredients:

- 4 tilapia fillets (about 1 lb total)
- 2 tbsp olive oil
- 2 tbsp freshly squeezed lemon juice
- 1 tsp grated lemon zest
- 1 tsp dried parsley
- 1/2 tsp garlic powder
- 1/4 tsp salt
- 1/4 tsp black pepper

Instructions:

1. Preheat the oven to 400°F. Lightly grease a baking dish or line with parchment paper.

2. In a small bowl, whisk together the olive oil, lemon juice, lemon zest, parsley, garlic powder, salt, and pepper.

3. Place the tilapia fillets in the prepared baking dish. Pour the lemon•herb mixture over the top, making sure to coat the fish evenly.

4. Bake for 12•15 minutes, or until the fish flakes easily with a fork and reaches an internal temperature of 145°F.

5. Serve the baked tilapia immediately, garnished with extra lemon wedges if desired. Enjoy!

The lemon and herb flavors complement the mild taste of the tilapia perfectly. This is a quick and easy baked fish recipe that's perfect for a healthy weeknight meal.

86. Shrimp Scampi (zucchini noodles)

Ingredients:

- 3 medium zucchinis, spiralized or julienned into noodles
- 1 lb large shrimp, peeled and deveined
- 3 tbsp unsalted butter
- 3 cloves garlic, minced
- 1/4 cup dry white wine
- 2 tbsp freshly squeezed lemon juice
- 2 tbsp chopped fresh parsley
- 1/4 tsp red pepper flakes (optional)
- Salt and pepper to taste
- Lemon wedges for serving

Instructions:

1. In a large skillet or sauté pan, melt the butter over medium heat. Add the minced garlic and cook for 1 minute until fragrant.

2. Add the shrimp to the pan and cook for 2•3 minutes per side, until the shrimp are opaque and cooked through. Transfer the shrimp to a plate and set aside.

3. Add the white wine and lemon juice to the pan. Bring the mixture to a simmer and cook for 2•3 minutes, scraping up any browned bits from the bottom of the pan.

4. Add the zucchini noodles to the pan and toss to coat them in the sauce. Cook for 2•3 minutes, just until the zucchini is tender but still crisp.

5. Remove the pan from heat and stir the cooked shrimp back into the zucchini noodles.

6. Sprinkle the chopped parsley and red pepper flakes (if using) over the top. Season with salt and pepper to taste.

7. Serve the shrimp scampi with zucchini noodles immediately, with lemon wedges on the side.

The zucchini noodles provide a low•carb, veggie•based alternative to traditional pasta in this shrimp scampi dish. The garlicky, lemony sauce coats the tender shrimp and zucchini perfectly.

This is a quick and easy healthy meal that's perfect for a weeknight dinner.

87. Hard•boiled Eggs

Ingredients:

• Large eggs

Instructions:

1. Place the eggs in a single layer in a saucepan and cover with cold water by 1 inch.

2. Bring the water to a boil over high heat. Once the water reaches a full boil, remove the pan from the heat and cover.

3. Let the eggs sit in the hot water for the following times, depending on your desired doneness:
• Soft•boiled: 6•7 minutes
• Hard•boiled: 12 minutes
• Extra hard•boiled: 15 minutes

4. Drain the hot water and cover the eggs with cold water. Let sit for 5 minutes.

5. Gently tap the eggs against the counter to crack the shells, then peel starting from the wider end of the egg.

6. Serve the hard•boiled eggs as is, or use them in recipes like deviled eggs, egg salad, or as a protein•packed snack.

Tips:
• Older eggs peel more easily than very fresh eggs.
• Adding a teaspoon of baking soda to the cooking water can also help with peeling.
• Store hard•boiled eggs in the refrigerator for up to 1 week.

Hard•boiled eggs are a versatile, protein•rich ingredient that can be enjoyed in many different ways. This simple method produces perfectly cooked eggs every time.

88. String Cheese

Ingredients:

- 1 gallon whole milk
- 1/4 teaspoon citric acid or 1/2 rennet tablet, dissolved in 1/4 cup water
- Salt (optional)

Instructions:

1. In a large pot, heat the milk over medium heat, stirring occasionally, until it reaches 185°F on a dairy thermometer.

2. Remove the pot from the heat and stir in the citric acid or dissolved rennet. The milk should start to curdle and form curds and whey.

3. Let the mixture sit for 5•10 minutes, until the curds have fully formed and separated from the whey.

4. Using a slotted spoon, scoop the curds out of the pot and into a colander to drain. Reserve the whey for other uses.

5. Knead the curds with your hands until they become smooth and stretchy, like mozzarella. You can add a pinch of salt at this stage if desired.

6. Divide the cheese into small pieces and stretch and pull them into long strings.

7. Place the string cheese pieces on a parchment•lined baking sheet and refrigerate for at least 2 hours before serving.

The string cheese can be stored in the refrigerator for up to 1 week. Enjoy!

89. Edamame

Ingredients:

- 1 lb fresh edamame in the pod
- 2 cups water
- 1 tbsp coarse sea salt or kosher salt

Instructions:

1. Bring the 2 cups of water to a boil in a medium saucepan.

2. Add the edamame pods and salt. Return to a boil.

3. Reduce heat and simmer for 5•7 minutes, until the pods are bright green and tender.

4. Drain the edamame in a colander and rinse with cold water to stop the cooking.

5. Serve the edamame warm or at room temperature, in the pods. Provide small bowls for the shells.

To eat, simply pick up a pod, place it in your mouth, and use your teeth to gently squeeze the beans out of the pod. Discard the empty pod.

You can also season the cooked edamame with additional salt, lemon juice, soy sauce, or other seasonings if desired. Edamame makes a great healthy snack or appetizer.

Enjoy your fresh, steamed edamame!

90. Apple Slices (with peanut butter)

Ingredients:

• 2 medium apples, cored and sliced
• 1/4 cup creamy peanut butter
• Optional toppings: cinnamon, honey, raisins, crushed nuts

Instructions:

1. Wash and core the apples. Slice them into thin, even slices, about 1/4 inch thick.

2. Arrange the apple slices on a plate or platter.

3. In a small bowl, stir the peanut butter until smooth and creamy.

4. Using a spoon or knife, spread a small amount of peanut butter onto each apple slice.

5. If desired, sprinkle the peanut butter•topped apple slices with any of the optional toppings:
• Cinnamon
• Drizzle of honey
• Raisins or other dried fruit
• Chopped nuts or seeds

6. Serve the apple slices with peanut butter immediately, or refrigerate until ready to serve.

This makes a simple, healthy, and delicious snack or light dessert. The peanut butter provides protein and healthy fats to balance out the natural sweetness of the apples.

You can use any type of apples you prefer, such as Gala, Fuji, or Honeycrisp. Adjust the amount of peanut butter to your taste. Enjoy!

91. Protein Bars (low•sugar)

Ingredients:

- 1 1/2 cups rolled oats
- 1 cup unsweetened shredded coconut
- 1/2 cup peanut butter (or other nut butter)
- 1/2 cup vanilla protein powder
- 1/4 cup honey or maple syrup
- 1/4 cup unsweetened applesauce
- 1 tsp vanilla extract
- 1/4 tsp salt

Optional add•ins:
- 1/4 cup chopped nuts or seeds
- 2 tbsp dark chocolate chips
- 1 tbsp chia or flax seeds

Instructions:

1. In a large bowl, mix together the rolled oats, shredded coconut, protein powder, and any optional add•ins.

2. In a separate bowl, whisk together the peanut butter, honey/maple syrup, applesauce, vanilla, and salt until well combined.

3. Pour the wet ingredients into the dry ingredients and stir until a thick, sticky dough forms.

4. Line an 8x8 inch baking pan with parchment paper. Press the dough evenly into the pan.

5. Refrigerate for at least 30 minutes to allow the bars to firm up.

6. Remove the bars from the pan and cut into 12 equal pieces.

7. Store the protein bars in an airtight container in the refrigerator for up to 1 week.

These low•sugar protein bars are a great healthy snack or on•the•go breakfast option. Adjust the sweetener and add•ins to your taste preferences.

92. Carrot Sticks (with hummus)

Ingredients:

• 4•5 medium carrots, peeled and cut into sticks
• 1 cup prepared hummus (store•bought or homemade)

Optional Toppings/Seasonings:
• Chopped fresh parsley or cilantro
• Paprika
• Crushed red pepper flakes
• Lemon wedges

Instructions:

1. Wash and peel the carrots. Cut them into long, thin sticks, about 4•5 inches long and 1/2 inch thick.

2. Place the carrot sticks in a bowl or on a plate.

3. Scoop the hummus into a small serving bowl or dish.

4. Arrange the carrot sticks around the hummus, allowing guests to dip the carrots into the hummus.

5. If desired, garnish the hummus with any of the optional toppings • chopped parsley/cilantro, paprika, crushed red pepper flakes, or a squeeze of fresh lemon juice.

That's it! This simple snack or appetizer is a great way to enjoy fresh, crunchy carrots with the creamy, protein•packed hummus.

The hummus provides a tasty dip for the carrots, making it a healthy and satisfying snack. You can use any flavor of hummus you prefer, such as classic, roasted red pepper, or garlic.

Enjoy your carrot sticks with hummus!

93. Cucumber Slices (with Greek yogurt dip)

Ingredients:

For the Dip:
• 1 cup plain Greek yogurt
• 2 tbsp fresh dill, chopped
• 1 tbsp lemon juice
• 1 garlic clove, minced
• 1/4 tsp salt
• 1/4 tsp black pepper

For the Cucumbers:
• 2 medium cucumbers, sliced into rounds

Instructions:

1. In a small bowl, mix together all the dip ingredients • Greek yogurt, dill, lemon juice, garlic, salt, and pepper. Stir until well combined.

2. Wash the cucumbers and slice them into 1/4•inch thick rounds.

3. Arrange the cucumber slices on a serving platter or plate.

4. Serve the Greek yogurt dip alongside the cucumber slices. You can either let guests dip the cucumbers into the dip, or you can spoon a small amount of dip onto each cucumber slice.

5. Refrigerate any leftover dip in an airtight container for up to 5 days.

The cool, crisp cucumbers pair perfectly with the tangy, herby Greek yogurt dip. This makes a refreshing and healthy snack or appetizer. You can adjust the seasonings in the dip to your taste preferences.

Enjoy your cucumber slices with this easy homemade Greek yogurt dip!

94. Celery Sticks (with light cream cheese)

Ingredients:

• 4•5 celery stalks, washed and cut into 3•4 inch sticks
• 4 oz light or reduced•fat cream cheese, softened
• Optional toppings: raisins, chopped nuts, dried cranberries, everything bagel seasoning

Instructions:

1. Wash the celery stalks and cut them into 3•4 inch sticks.

2. In a small bowl, use a spoon or small spatula to spread a thin layer of the softened light cream cheese onto one side of each celery stick.

3. If desired, top the cream cheese•filled celery sticks with any of the optional toppings, such as:
• Raisins
• Chopped walnuts, almonds, or pecans
• Dried cranberries
• Everything bagel seasoning

4. Arrange the filled celery sticks on a plate or platter and serve immediately.

This makes a simple, healthy, and tasty snack or appetizer. The crunchy celery pairs perfectly with the creamy, tangy light cream cheese.

The optional toppings add extra flavor, texture, and nutrition. The raisins or dried cranberries provide natural sweetness, while the nuts add a satisfying crunch.

You can prepare the celery sticks and cream cheese filling in advance and assemble them just before serving. Store any leftover filled celery sticks in an airtight container in the refrigerator for up to 3•4 days.

Enjoy these easy and delicious celery sticks with light cream cheese!

95. Turkey Roll•ups (with light cheese)

Ingredients:

- 8 slices deli•style turkey breast
- 4 slices light/low•fat cheddar or Swiss cheese, halved
- Dijon mustard (optional)

Instructions:

1. Lay the turkey slices out flat on a clean work surface.

2. Place a half•slice of cheese near the center of each turkey slice.

3. If desired, spread a small amount of Dijon mustard over the cheese.

4. Carefully roll up the turkey slice around the cheese, tucking in the sides as you go.

5. Secure the roll•up with a toothpick or small skewer, if needed.

6. Repeat with the remaining turkey and cheese slices.

7. Serve the turkey roll•ups immediately, or refrigerate until ready to serve.

These turkey roll•ups make a quick, easy, and healthy snack or light meal. The combination of lean turkey and light cheese provides protein and flavor.

You can customize the fillings by using different types of cheese, such as provolone or pepper jack. You can also add other ingredients like sliced avocado, roasted red peppers, or a drizzle of balsamic glaze.

For a heartier option, you can serve the turkey roll•ups with whole grain crackers, sliced vegetables, or a small side salad.

Store any leftover roll•ups in an airtight container in the refrigerator for up to 3•4 days.

Enjoy these simple and delicious turkey roll•ups with light cheese!

96. Greek Yogurt (with honey)

Ingredients:

• 32 oz (4 cups) plain Greek yogurt
• 2•4 tablespoons honey, to taste

Instructions:

1. Scoop the Greek yogurt into a serving bowl or individual bowls.

2. Drizzle the honey over the top of the yogurt, using 2•4 tablespoons depending on how sweet you want it.

3. Gently stir the honey into the yogurt until it is well combined.

4. Serve immediately or refrigerate until ready to enjoy.

Tips:
• Use full•fat or 2% Greek yogurt for a richer, creamier texture.

• Try different types of honey like clover, wildflower or raw honey for variety.

• Top with fresh fruit, granola, nuts or a sprinkle of cinnamon if desired.

• This makes a great healthy breakfast, snack or dessert.

97. Protein Muffins

Ingredients:

- 1 cup oat flour (or whole wheat flour)
- 1/2 cup vanilla protein powder
- 1 tsp baking powder
- 1/4 tsp salt
- 1/2 cup unsweetened applesauce
- 1/4 cup honey or maple syrup
- 1/4 cup unsweetened almond milk
- 2 large eggs
- 1 tsp vanilla extract

Optional Mix•Ins:
- 1/2 cup blueberries, raspberries, or chopped nuts
- 2 tbsp chia or flax seeds
- 1/4 cup dark chocolate chips

Instructions:
1. Preheat your oven to 350°F (175°C). Grease a 12•cup muffin tin or line with paper liners.

2. In a medium bowl, whisk together the oat flour, protein powder, baking powder, and salt.

3. In a separate bowl, combine the applesauce, honey/maple syrup, almond milk, eggs, and vanilla. Mix well.

4. Pour the wet ingredients into the dry ingredients and stir just until combined. Do not overmix.

5. Fold in any desired mix•ins, such as berries, nuts, chia/flax seeds, or chocolate chips.

6. Divide the batter evenly among the prepared muffin cups, filling them about 3/4 full.

7. Bake for 18•22 minutes, or until a toothpick inserted in the center comes out clean.

8. Allow the muffins to cool in the tin for 5 minutes before transferring them to a wire rack to cool completely.

These protein•packed muffins make a great healthy breakfast, snack, or on•the•go option. The protein powder, eggs, and optional mix•ins provide a boost of protein and nutrients.

Store the muffins in an airtight container at room temperature for up to 4 days, or freeze for longer storage.

98. Roasted Chickpeas

Ingredients:

- 1 (15 oz) can chickpeas (garbanzo beans), drained and rinsed
- 1 tbsp olive oil
- 1 tsp ground cumin
- 1 tsp paprika
- 1/2 tsp garlic powder
- 1/4 tsp salt
- 1/4 tsp black pepper

Instructions:

1. Preheat your oven to 400°F (200°C).

2. Drain and rinse the chickpeas, then pat them dry thoroughly with paper towels or a clean kitchen towel.

3. In a medium bowl, toss the chickpeas with the olive oil, cumin, paprika, garlic powder, salt, and black pepper until they are evenly coated.

4. Spread the seasoned chickpeas out in a single layer on a baking sheet lined with parchment paper.

5. Roast the chickpeas for 20•25 minutes, stirring halfway, until they are crispy and golden brown.

6. Remove the roasted chickpeas from the oven and let them cool for 5 minutes before serving.

You can enjoy the roasted chickpeas as a snack on their own, or use them as a topping for salads, soups, or grain bowls. They make a great crunchy, protein•packed alternative to nuts or crackers.

For different flavor variations, try using other spice blends like chili powder, curry powder, or Italian seasoning. You can also toss the roasted chickpeas with a bit of honey or maple syrup for a sweet•and•savory treat.

Store any leftover roasted chickpeas in an airtight container at room temperature for up to 1 week.

Enjoy your crispy, flavorful roasted chickpeas!

99. Pumpkin Seeds

Ingredients:

- 1 cup raw pumpkin seeds (also called pepitas)
- 1 tbsp olive oil or melted coconut oil
- 1 tsp salt (or more to taste)
- Optional seasonings: garlic powder, onion powder, chili powder, cumin, etc.

Instructions:

1. Preheat your oven to 325°F (165°C).

2. Rinse the pumpkin seeds under cold water to remove any pulp or strings. Pat them dry completely with paper towels or a clean kitchen towel.

3. In a small bowl, toss the clean, dry pumpkin seeds with the olive or coconut oil until they are evenly coated.

4. Spread the oiled seeds out in a single layer on a baking sheet lined with parchment paper.

5. Sprinkle the salt (and any other desired seasonings) evenly over the seeds.

6. Roast the pumpkin seeds for 18•22 minutes, stirring halfway, until they are lightly golden brown.

7. Remove the roasted pumpkin seeds from the oven and let them cool completely before serving.

The seeds can be stored in an airtight container at room temperature for up to 1 week.

Pumpkin seeds make a great healthy snack, packed with protein, fiber, healthy fats, and various vitamins and minerals. Adjust the seasoning to your taste preferences. Enjoy your freshly roasted pumpkin seeds!

100. Sunflower Seeds

Ingredients:

- 1 cup raw, shelled sunflower seeds
- 1 tablespoon olive oil or melted coconut oil
- 1 teaspoon salt (or more to taste)
- Optional seasonings: garlic powder, onion powder, paprika, chili powder, etc.

Instructions:

1. Preheat your oven to 325°F (165°C).

2. In a small bowl, toss the raw sunflower seeds with the olive or coconut oil until they are evenly coated.

3. Spread the oiled sunflower seeds out in a single layer on a baking sheet lined with parchment paper.

4. Sprinkle the salt (and any other desired seasonings) evenly over the seeds.

5. Roast the sunflower seeds for 15•20 minutes, stirring halfway, until they are lightly golden brown.

6. Remove the roasted sunflower seeds from the oven and let them cool completely before serving.

The seeds can be stored in an airtight container at room temperature for up to 2 weeks.

Roasted sunflower seeds make a great healthy snack, packed with protein, healthy fats, fiber, and various vitamins and minerals. Adjust the seasoning to your taste preferences. You can also try different flavor combinations, like chili lime or garlic parmesan.

Enjoy your freshly roasted sunflower seeds!

101. Almonds (unsalted)

Ingredients:

• 1 cup raw, unsalted almonds

Instructions:

1. Measure out 1 cup of raw, unsalted almonds.

2. You can enjoy the almonds as•is, straight from the bag or container. No further preparation is needed.

That's it! Unsalted almonds make a great healthy snack option.

Some tips for enjoying unsalted almonds:

• Portion control is key, as almonds are high in calories and fat, even though they are healthy fats. Stick to a 1/4 or 1/2 cup serving.

• You can store the almonds in an airtight container at room temperature for up to 2 weeks.

• For extra flavor, you can toast the almonds in a dry skillet over medium heat for 2•3 minutes, stirring frequently, until fragrant.

• Try pairing the unsalted almonds with other healthy snacks like fresh fruit, Greek yogurt, or a small piece of dark chocolate.

The unsalted almonds provide a satisfying crunch and are packed with protein, fiber, healthy fats, vitamins, and minerals. They make a great portable, nutrient•dense snack.

Enjoy your unsalted almonds as a healthy, delicious treat!

102. Mixed Berries

Ingredients:

- 1 cup fresh blueberries
- 1 cup fresh raspberries
- 1 cup fresh blackberries
- 1 cup fresh strawberries, hulled and halved

Instructions:

1. Gently rinse the berries under cool running water and pat them dry with a paper towel or clean kitchen towel.

2. In a large bowl, combine the blueberries, raspberries, blackberries, and strawberries. Gently toss the berries together.

3. Serve the mixed berries immediately, or refrigerate until ready to enjoy.

That's it! This is a simple, healthy, and delicious snack or side dish.

The combination of different types of berries provides a variety of flavors, textures, and nutritional benefits. Berries are packed with antioxidants, fiber, vitamins, and minerals.

You can enjoy the mixed berries as is, or try topping them with a light drizzle of honey, a sprinkle of chopped nuts, or a dollop of Greek yogurt for added flavor and nutrition.

The mixed berries can also be used in smoothies, salads, oatmeal, or as a topping for pancakes or waffles.

Store any leftover mixed berries in the refrigerator for up to 5 days.

Enjoy this refreshing and nutritious mixed berry snack!

103. Bell Pepper Slices (with hummus)

Ingredients:

- 1•2 bell peppers (any color), washed and sliced into strips
- 1 cup prepared hummus (store•bought or homemade)

Optional Toppings/Seasonings:
- Chopped fresh parsley or cilantro
- Paprika
- Crushed red pepper flakes
- Lemon wedges

Instructions:

1. Wash the bell peppers and slice them into long, thin strips, about 1/2 inch thick.

2. Arrange the bell pepper slices on a serving platter or plate.

3. Scoop the hummus into a small bowl or dish and place it in the center of the plate with the bell pepper slices around it.

4. If desired, garnish the hummus with any of the optional toppings • chopped parsley or cilantro, a sprinkle of paprika, crushed red pepper flakes, or a squeeze of fresh lemon juice.

That's it! This simple snack or appetizer is a great way to enjoy fresh, crunchy bell peppers with the creamy, protein•packed hummus.

The hummus provides a tasty dip for the bell pepper slices, making it a healthy and satisfying snack. You can use any flavor of hummus you prefer, such as classic, roasted red pepper, or garlic.

Enjoy your bell pepper slices with hummus!

104. Low•fat Cottage Cheese (with fruit)

Ingredients:

• 1 cup low•fat or non•fat cottage cheese
• 1/2 cup fresh fruit (such as berries, diced apple, mango, etc.)
• 1•2 teaspoons honey or maple syrup (optional)

Instructions:

1. Scoop the cottage cheese into a small bowl or container.

2. Top the cottage cheese with your choice of fresh fruit. Some great options include:
• Blueberries, raspberries, or strawberries
• Diced apple, pear, or peach
• Mango or pineapple chunks
• Sliced bananas

3. If desired, drizzle 1•2 teaspoons of honey or maple syrup over the top of the fruit and cottage cheese.

4. Gently stir the fruit and sweetener (if using) into the cottage cheese until well combined.

5. Serve immediately or refrigerate until ready to enjoy.

This makes a quick, healthy, and satisfying snack or light breakfast. The cottage cheese provides protein, while the fruit adds natural sweetness, fiber, and vitamins.

You can use any type of fresh fruit that you enjoy. Berries, stone fruits, and tropical fruits all pair well with the creamy cottage cheese.

Feel free to adjust the amount of sweetener to your taste preferences. Some people find the cottage cheese is sweet enough on its own when paired with the fruit.

Enjoy your low•fat cottage cheese with fresh fruit!

105. Avocado Toast (whole grain)

Ingredients:

- 2 slices whole grain or multigrain bread
- 1 ripe avocado, halved and pitted
- 1 tbsp olive oil or avocado oil
- 1 tsp lemon juice
- 1/4 tsp salt
- 1/4 tsp black pepper
- Optional toppings: sliced tomatoes, sprouts, red pepper flakes, everything bagel seasoning

Instructions:

1. Toast the whole grain bread slices until lightly golden brown.

2. In a small bowl, mash the avocado flesh with a fork until it reaches your desired consistency (chunky or smooth).

3. Add the olive or avocado oil, lemon juice, salt, and black pepper to the mashed avocado. Stir to combine.

4. Spread the avocado mixture evenly over the toasted bread slices.

5. Top the avocado toast with any desired additional toppings, such as sliced tomatoes, sprouts, a sprinkle of red pepper flakes, or everything bagel seasoning.

6. Serve the avocado toast immediately.

The whole grain bread provides complex carbs, fiber, and nutrients, while the avocado adds healthy fats, vitamins, and creaminess. This makes a satisfying and nutritious breakfast, snack, or light meal.

You can customize the toppings to your liking. The possibilities are endless for delicious and healthy avocado toast variations.

Enjoy your avocado toast on wholesome whole grain bread!

106. Greek Yogurt (with cocoa powder)

Ingredients:

• 1 cup plain Greek yogurt
• 1•2 tablespoons unsweetened cocoa powder
• 1•2 teaspoons honey or maple syrup (optional)

Instructions:

1. In a small bowl, add the plain Greek yogurt.

2. Sprinkle the unsweetened cocoa powder over the yogurt and stir to combine. Start with 1 tablespoon of cocoa powder and add more to taste.

3. If you want it a bit sweeter, drizzle in 1•2 teaspoons of honey or maple syrup and stir again until well mixed.

4. Serve immediately or refrigerate until ready to enjoy.

That's it! This simple recipe turns plain Greek yogurt into a delicious, chocolatey treat.

The Greek yogurt provides protein, probiotics, and creaminess, while the cocoa powder adds a rich chocolate flavor. The optional honey or maple syrup can provide a touch of sweetness if desired.

This makes a great healthy snack or light dessert. You can also top it with fresh berries, chopped nuts, or a sprinkle of cinnamon for extra flavor and nutrition.

Enjoy your Greek yogurt with cocoa powder!

107. Protein Ice Cream

Ingredients:

- 1 cup plain Greek yogurt
- 1 scoop (about 30g) vanilla or unflavored protein powder
- 1/4 cup unsweetened almond milk (or milk of your choice)
- 1•2 tbsp honey or maple syrup (optional)
- 1/2 tsp vanilla extract
- Pinch of salt

Optional Mix•Ins:
- Cocoa powder
- Peanut butter
- Berries
- Chopped nuts
- Chocolate chips

Instructions:

1. In a medium bowl, combine the Greek yogurt, protein powder, almond milk, honey/maple syrup (if using), vanilla extract, and salt. Whisk or stir until the mixture is smooth and well combined.

2. If desired, fold in any of the optional mix•ins, such as cocoa powder, peanut butter, berries, chopped nuts, or chocolate chips.

3. Pour the mixture into a shallow baking dish or freezer•safe container.

4. Cover and freeze for 2•3 hours, stirring and scraping the sides every 30 minutes, until the ice cream reaches your desired consistency.

5. Scoop and serve the protein ice cream immediately, or transfer to an airtight container and freeze for up to 2 weeks.

The Greek yogurt and protein powder provide a boost of protein, while the almond milk and optional sweeteners create a creamy, ice cream•like texture. Adjust the amount of sweetener to your taste preferences.

This high•protein ice cream makes a great healthy dessert or snack. Enjoy it on its own or with your favorite toppings!

108. Baked Apples (with cinnamon)

Ingredients:

• 4 medium•sized apples (such as Gala, Honeycrisp, or Fuji)
• 2 tablespoons brown sugar
• 1 teaspoon ground cinnamon
• 2 tablespoons unsalted butter, cubed
• 1/4 cup water or apple cider

Optional Toppings:
• Vanilla ice cream or whipped cream
• Chopped walnuts or pecans
• Caramel sauce

Instructions:

1. Preheat your oven to 375°F (190°C).

2. Wash and core the apples, leaving a small well in the center of each one. Place the apples in a baking dish.

3. In a small bowl, mix together the brown sugar and cinnamon. Spoon this mixture into the center of each apple, dividing it evenly.

4. Top each apple with a small cube of butter.

5. Pour the water or apple cider into the bottom of the baking dish, being careful not to pour it over the apples.

6. Bake the apples for 30•40 minutes, or until they are tender when pierced with a fork. The skins should be wrinkled, and the filling should be bubbly.

7. Remove the baked apples from the oven and let them cool for 5•10 minutes.

8. Serve the baked apples warm, with any desired toppings like vanilla ice cream, whipped cream, chopped nuts, or caramel sauce.

The baked apples will be soft and tender, with a sweet, cinnamon•spiced filling. This makes a delicious and healthy dessert or snack.

Enjoy your homemade baked apples with cinnamon!

109. Chia Seed Pudding (with vanilla)

Ingredients:

- 1 cup unsweetened almond milk (or milk of your choice)
- 3 tbsp chia seeds
- 1 tsp vanilla extract
- 1•2 tsp honey or maple syrup (optional)

Instructions:

1. In a medium bowl or mason jar, whisk together the almond milk, chia seeds, and vanilla extract until well combined.

2. If you want the pudding to be a bit sweeter, stir in 1•2 teaspoons of honey or maple syrup.

3. Cover the bowl or seal the mason jar and refrigerate for at least 2 hours, or overnight. The chia seeds will thicken the mixture into a pudding•like consistency.

4. Once the chia pudding has set, give it a good stir to break up any clumps.

5. Serve the vanilla chia pudding chilled, either on its own or topped with:
- Fresh berries
- Sliced bananas or other fruit
- Chopped nuts or toasted coconut
- A drizzle of nut butter

This chia seed pudding is a nutritious, protein•packed, and delicious breakfast, snack, or dessert. The vanilla flavor pairs perfectly with the natural sweetness of the chia seeds.

You can make this recipe in advance and keep it refrigerated for up to 5 days. Adjust the amount of sweetener to your taste preferences.

Enjoy your homemade vanilla chia seed pudding!

110. Sugar•free Popsicles

Ingredients:

• 2 cups unsweetened fruit puree (such as mashed bananas, applesauce, or blended berries)
• 1/4 cup unsweetened almond milk or coconut milk
• 1•2 tbsp zero•calorie sweetener (like stevia, erythritol, or monk fruit)
• 1 tsp vanilla extract (optional)

Instructions:

1. In a medium bowl, mix together the fruit puree, milk, sweetener, and vanilla (if using) until well combined.

2. Carefully pour the mixture into popsicle molds, leaving a little room at the top for expansion.

3. Insert popsicle sticks into the center of each mold.

4. Freeze the popsicles for at least 4•6 hours, or until completely frozen.

5. To remove the popsicles, run the molds under warm water for 30 seconds to 1 minute, then gently pull the popsicles out.

Flavor Variations:
• Strawberry: Use pureed fresh or frozen strawberries
• Mango: Use pureed fresh or frozen mango
• Chocolate: Add 2•3 tbsp unsweetened cocoa powder
• Creamy Vanilla: Use plain Greek yogurt instead of fruit puree

These sugar•free popsicles are a healthy, refreshing treat. The fruit puree provides natural sweetness, while the milk adds creaminess. The zero•calorie sweetener can be adjusted to your taste preferences.

Store any leftover popsicles in the freezer for up to 2 months. Enjoy these easy, guilt•free popsicles!

Congratulations on completing the *Gastric Bypass Meal Prep Cookbook: 110+ Prep-Ready Recipes for a Healthier You.* We hope this collection of recipes has provided you with the tools, inspiration, and confidence to take control of your nutrition and achieve lasting success in your health journey.

Reflecting on Your Journey

Adapting to life after gastric bypass surgery is a transformative experience that requires dedication, resilience, and a commitment to new dietary habits. Meal prepping has been shown to be an invaluable strategy for managing your nutritional needs and ensuring that you stay on track with your health goals. By planning and preparing your meals in advance, you have taken a proactive step towards a healthier, more balanced lifestyle.

Key Takeaways

- *Nutrient-Dense Meals*: Each recipe in this cookbook has been designed to provide you with the essential nutrients your body needs, focusing on high-protein, low-fat, and easily digestible ingredients.

- *Convenience and Consistency:* Meal prepping simplifies your daily routine, allowing you to enjoy nutritious, delicious meals without the stress of last-minute cooking. This consistency is crucial for maintaining your dietary plan and achieving long-term success.

- *Portion Control and Mindful Eating:* By prepping your meals in advance, you can better manage portion sizes and ensure that each meal aligns with your post-surgery dietary requirements. This helps prevent overeating and supports mindful eating habits.

Moving Forward

As you continue on your journey, remember that meal prepping is not just a short-term solution but a sustainable lifestyle choice. Continue to explore new recipes, experiment with different ingredients, and find joy in the process of preparing meals that nourish your body and support your health goals.

Thank you for allowing us to be a part of your journey. Here's to your continued health, happiness, and culinary adventures. May your meals always be nourishing, satisfying, and a testament to your commitment to a healthier lifestyle.

Happy prepping and bon appétit!